Marcel Werner Stahl

Cellular prion protein (PrPC) in Caenorhabditis elegans

Marcel Werner Stahl

Cellular prion protein (PrPC) in Caenorhabditis elegans

Investigation of the physiologic function of human prion protein in a new model organism

Südwestdeutscher Verlag für Hochschulschriften

Impressum/Imprint (nur für Deutschland/only for Germany)
Bibliografische Information der Deutschen Nationalbibliothek: Die Deutsche Nationalbibliothek verzeichnet diese Publikation in der Deutschen Nationalbibliografie; detaillierte bibliografische Daten sind im Internet über http://dnb.d-nb.de abrufbar.
Alle in diesem Buch genannten Marken und Produktnamen unterliegen warenzeichen-, marken- oder patentrechtlichem Schutz bzw. sind Warenzeichen oder eingetragene Warenzeichen der jeweiligen Inhaber. Die Wiedergabe von Marken, Produktnamen, Gebrauchsnamen, Handelsnamen, Warenbezeichnungen u.s.w. in diesem Werk berechtigt auch ohne besondere Kennzeichnung nicht zu der Annahme, dass solche Namen im Sinne der Warenzeichen- und Markenschutzgesetzgebung als frei zu betrachten wären und daher von jedermann benutzt werden dürften.

Verlag: Südwestdeutscher Verlag für Hochschulschriften GmbH & Co. KG
Heinrich-Böcking-Str. 6-8, 66121 Saarbrücken, Deutschland
Telefon +49 681 37 20 271-1, Telefax +49 681 37 20 271-0
Email: info@svh-verlag.de

Approved by: Ulm, Universität Ulm, Dissertation, 2010

Herstellung in Deutschland:
Schaltungsdienst Lange o.H.G., Berlin
Books on Demand GmbH, Norderstedt
Reha GmbH, Saarbrücken
Amazon Distribution GmbH, Leipzig
ISBN: 978-3-8381-2506-0

Imprint (only for USA, GB)
Bibliographic information published by the Deutsche Nationalbibliothek: The Deutsche Nationalbibliothek lists this publication in the Deutsche Nationalbibliografie; detailed bibliographic data are available in the Internet at http://dnb.d-nb.de.
Any brand names and product names mentioned in this book are subject to trademark, brand or patent protection and are trademarks or registered trademarks of their respective holders. The use of brand names, product names, common names, trade names, product descriptions etc. even without a particular marking in this works is in no way to be construed to mean that such names may be regarded as unrestricted in respect of trademark and brand protection legislation and could thus be used by anyone.

Publisher: Südwestdeutscher Verlag für Hochschulschriften GmbH & Co. KG
Heinrich-Böcking-Str. 6-8, 66121 Saarbrücken, Germany
Phone +49 681 37 20 271-1, Fax +49 681 37 20 271-0
Email: info@svh-verlag.de

Printed in the U.S.A.
Printed in the U.K. by (see last page)
ISBN: 978-3-8381-2506-0

Copyright © 2012 by the author and Südwestdeutscher Verlag für Hochschulschriften GmbH & Co. KG and licensors
All rights reserved. Saarbrücken 2012

*In memory of my friend Florian Brenner,
You will never be forgotten.*

Index of contents

		List of abbreviations	IV
1		Introduction	1
	1.1	Historical approach to the prion protein	1
	1.2	The physiological function of PrP^C	5
	1.3	*Caenorhabditis elegans*	15
	1.4	Objective of this work	19
2		Material and methods	20
	2.1	Material	20
	2.2	Methods	26
3		Results	43
	3.1	GFP fluorescence	43
	3.2	Western blot	47
	3.3	Lifespan determination	49
	3.4	Paraquat stress assays	58
	3.5	Heat stress assays	75
	3.6	Copper stress assay	80
	3.7	Paraquat stress assay after previous Cu^{2+} treatment	82
	3.8	Hydrogen peroxide stress assay	84
	3.9	SOD enzyme assay	87
	3.10	Dye fill	89
4		Discussion	92
	4.1	Verification of the obtained data	92
	4.2	PrP^C involved in oxidative stress response	93
	4.3	PrP^C and its role in natural lifespan	103
	4.4	Conclusion and outlook	105
5		Summary	107
6		Literature	109

List of abbreviations

aa	Amino acid
abu-11	Activated gene in Blocked Unfolded protein response
AD	Alzheimer's disease
AFD	Thermosensory neuron
age-1	Ageing alteration gene
APP	Amyloid precursor protein
AQR	Special chemosensory neuron
Bak	Bcl-2 antagonist killer
BamHI	Restriction endnuclease Bacillus amyloliquefaciens H
Bax	Bcl-2 associated X-protein
BCA	Bicinchoninic acid
Bcl-2	B-cell lymphoma 2
BH3	Bcl-2 homology domain 3
BSA	Bovine serum albumine
C. elegans	*Caenorhabditis elegans*
cm	Centimeter(s)
CNS	Central nervous system
conc.	Concentration
CWD	Chronic Wasting Disease
ddH$_2$O	Double-Distilled water
DAF (*daf*)	Abnormal Dauer formation
DAPi	4',6-Diamidino-2-phenylindol
DiI	Fluorescent dye
Dpl	Doppel gene
E. coli	*Escherichia coli*
EcoRI	Nuclease I out *E. coli* tribe R
ER	Endoplasmatic Recticulum
ERK	Extracellular-signal regulated kinase
ELISA	Enzyme-linked immunosorbent assay
Euk	SOD mimetic
fCJD	Familial Creutzfeldt-Jakob-Disease
FDUR	5-fluoro-2'-deoxyuridine

List of abbreviations

FFI	Fatal familial insomnia
FSI	Fatal sporadic insomnia
Fyn	Fyn tyrosine kinase
g	Gramm
GFP	Green fluorescent protein
GPI	Glycophosphatidylinositol
GSS	Gerstmann-Sträussler-Scheinker
Grb2	Growth factor receptor-bound protein 2
h	Hour(s)
HSF	Heat Shock Factor
HSP	Heat Shock Protein
IIS	Insulin/insulin-like signalling
Inhib.	Inhibitory
IPTG	Isopropyl-β-D-thiogalactopyranosid
ISP-1	Iron sulfor protein
JNK1/2	C-Jun N-terminal kinases 1/2
kDa	Kilo Dalton (1 Da = 1 u)
KpnI	Restriction endonuclease Klebsiella pneumonia
L	Liter(s)
L1, L2, L3, L4	*C. elegans* larval stages
MAPK	Mitogen-activated protein kinase
MBM	Meat and bone meal
MCF-7	Human breast adenocarcinoma cell line
MEK/MKK	see MAPK
min	Minute(s)
ml	Millilitre(s)
mm	Millimetre(s)
µg	Microgram(s)
N2a	Neuroblastoma cells
NCAM	Neural cell adhesion molecule
ng	Nano gram
NGM	Nematode growth medium
NADPH	Nicotinamide adenine dinucleotide phosphate

List of abbreviations

NFκB	Nuclear factor kappa-light-chain-enhancer of activated B cells
OP 50	*Escherichia coli* strain
otv	Of total volume
p38	Protein 38
p53	Protein 53
PAP	Peroxidase Anti-Peroxidase
PBS	Phosphate buffering saline
PCR	Polymerase Chain Reaction
pEGFP	Vector (Plasmid)
pha-1	Defective pharynx development
PKA, PKB	Protein kinase A, B
PMSF	Phenylmethylsulfonylfluorid
PQ^{2+}	Paraquat
$PQ^{\cdot-}$	Paraquat radical
PQR	Special chemosensory neuron
prnp	Prion protein gene
$Prn-p^{0/0}$	Prion protein gene homozygous lacking
PrP^C	Cellular protease resistant protein
PrP^{Sc}	Protease resistant prion protein
$PrP^{0/0}$	Prion protein deficient
PrPΔN	Prion protein lacking residues 32-121
Psel-12	P-selectin-12
recPrP	Recombinant prion protein
ROS	Reactive oxygen species
rpm	Rounds per minute
RS	Reactive species
RT	Room temperature
s	Second(s)
SAPK	Stress activated protein kinase
SDS-PAGE	Sodium dodecyl sulfate polyacrylamide gel electrophoresis
sel-12	Suppressor/Enhancer gene of Lin12
SIR-2.1	Member of the Sirtuin family

List of abbreviations

SKN-1/Nrf-2	SKiNhead transcription factor
SmaI	Restriction endonuclease
Src	Sarcoma cellular kinase
stand.	Standard
STI1	Stress-inducible protein 1
SOD	Superoxide Dismutase
t	Time
TBS	Tris-buffered saline
TCR	T cell receptor
Tg mice	Transgenic mice
TME	Transmissible mink encephalopathy
TNFα	Tumor necrosis factor α
TSE	Transmissible spongiform encephalopathy
U	Units
UV	Ultraviolet
wtPrP	Wildtype prion protein
6H4	Mouse monoclonal antibody against prion protein

1 Introduction

1.1 Historical approach to the prion protein

1.1.1 The first clinical description

It was in 1920 when the German neuropathologist Hans Gerhard Creutzfeldt (1885-1964) first published material, describing a clinical picture and a pathologic process now known as Creutzfeldt-Jakob disease (CJD). He thereby beat Alfons Maria Jakob's publication, a German neurologist (1884-1931), about the same syndrome by half a year. While CJD is the most famous member of prion protein diseases [152], it was Josef Gerstmann (1887-1969), an Austrian Professor in Neurology and Psychiatry [204], that first described a syndrome which is now a member of the prion protein diseases as well, the Gerstmann-Sträussler-Scheinker (GSS) disease. It was in 1924 when Gerstmann started to describe this syndrome, mainly impressed by a new unknown cause of finger agnosia and disorientation [72], until in 1936 he characterized it in its whole entity by cerebellar ataxia, slurred speech, pyramidal tract signs, ophthalmoplegia, features of dementia and parkinsonism [73]. In 1930, the first evidence was found regarding the inheritable aspect of CJD when a high incidence of CJD in certain families was shown, distinguishing sporadic CJD from familial (f)CJD [131, 190]. The clustering affect of CJD was resumed, especially in the 70's and 80's, where attempts were made to identify the origin and way of transmission of CJD in epidemiologic studies. Most famously, it was recorded that Libyan Jews had a 30 fold higher risk of coming down with CJD then other descending Israelis [103].

Over the years more and more similar syndromes were described in humans and other mammals (table 1), although at the time of discovery it was not known to be transmissible and infectious, or even interconnected. It was not until 1954 that Bjorn Sigurdsson first recognized a transmissible pattern in scrapie sheep and suggested an infection by a slow latent virus [179]. This was followed five years later by the insight that Kuru was connected to scrapie as well as to CJD [78, 108]. Still, it took until 1966 for Gajdusek to be able to prove transmission of Kuru-like symptoms in chimpanzees by inoculation [71]. It was then, in 1978, that Masters showed a variable spongiform degeneration and correlating reactive gliosis when the term transmissible spongiform encephalitis was derived [127].

Tab. 1: List of prion protein diseases (adopted from Prusiner [152])
iCJD, iatrogenic CJD; vCJD, variant CJD; fCJD, familial CJD; sCJD, sporadic CJD; GSS, Gerstmann–Sträussler–Sheinker disease; FFI, fatal familial insomnia; FSI, fatal sporadic insomnia; BSE, bovine spongiform encephalopathy; TME, transmissible mink encephalopathy; CWD, chronic wasting disease; FSE, feline spongiform encephalopathy; MBM, meat and bone meal.

Disease	Host	Mechanism of pathogenesis
Kuru	Fore people	Infection through ritualistic cannibalism
fCJD	Humans	Germ-line mutations in PrP gene
vCJD, nvCJD	Humans	Infection from bovine prion proteins
iCJD	Humans	Infection from prion-contaminated grafts
sCJD	Humans	Somatic mutation or spontaneous conversion of PrP^C to PrP^{Sc}
FFI	Humans	Germ-line mutations in PrP gene
GSS	Humans	Germ-line mutations in PrP gene
FSI	Humans	Somatic mutation or spontaneous conversion of PrP^C to PrP^{Sc} ?
Scrapie	Sheep	Infection in genetically susceptible sheep
BSE	Cattle	Infection with prion-contaminated MBM
TME	Mink	Infection with prion from sheep or cattle
CWD	Mule deer, elk	unknown
FSE	Cats	Infection with prion-contaminated bovine tissues or MBM
Exotic ungulate encephalopathy	Kulu, nyala, oryx	Infection with prion-contaminated MBM

1.1.2 Development of the prion protein theory

While most research focused on identifying a viral pathogen as the underlying cause, with other research fitting into the unquestioned theory of nucleic acid being an absolute requirement for being an infectious trigger, it was Stanley Ben Prusiner in 1972, who, at the start of his residency in neurology at the University of California San Francisco, was fascinated by a female patient dying of

Introduction

CJD just two months after disease onset, her brain being destroyed while her body remained unaffected by this process. She did not show any febrile response, no leukocytosis or pleocytosis, nor humoral immune response, although she was told that she was infected with a slow virus [152]. Ten years after Prusiner started research, he announced, in 1982, the idea of a protein, the prion protein (PrP), being the main part of the infectious agent [150], describing it in more detail in 1991 [151] as the physiological or cellular PrP^C which changesits secondary structure from 40% α-helix and to a little extent β-sheet to PrP^{Sc} consisting of 30% α-helix and to 45% β-sheet [144].

His discovery was preceded by years of sedimentation trials in an attempt to purify the scrapie agent with which he infected mice by inoculation, sacrificing the same after 120 days, when he thought the infectious titre was at its highest point, and he sedimented the mice's brain and spleen with different gradients to let new mice inoculate to the specific supernatant to check if it was still infectious, which took one year to manifest in the mice. This research was a large step forward, as it was discovered that Syrian Hamsters only needed 70 days to manifest the disease, and it also simplified endpoint titration, speeding up the trial by a factor of 100 [152].

After finding the right sediment, he was already puzzled by a finding of Alper in 1966, who documented that the so far smallest known viruses, the single stranded DNA phages ΦX174 and S13 as well as the RNA phages, needed just one tenth the level of irradiation to disintegrate than did the scrapie agent, leaving a size less then 800 bases, from which he concluded that this agent must be of unusual nature [4]. Prusiner was able to affirm these findings by showing that the infectious scrapie agent was sensitive to protein modifying procedures like hyrdolyzation but resistant to procedures modifying nucleic acids [153]. This was followed by the breakthrough of Prusiner and his colleague Bolton in 1984, in which the first structural component of the prion protein, the PrP 27-30, was identified [21] [155]. This also proved to be unique to the infectious prion protein, since it showed to be partly resistant to digestion by proteinase K, a quality shared only by prion protein found in scrapie infected tissues, and not by prion protein found in healthy uninfected animals [142]. Therefore the term PrP^C, for the normal variant, and PrP^{Sc}, for the infectious variant, derived, with both having 209 residues, but in PrP^{Sc} proteinase K just being able to cleave of the N-terminus, leaving 142 amino acids with a molecular weight of 27-30 kDa therefore called PrP 27-30 [133]. The term "Prion protein", on the other hand, was a Prusiner's mixture of the terms "PROteinaceous" and "INfectious", and denotes the infectious agent, while PrP stands for "Proteinase resistant Protein" [150], but is also used as an acronym for prion protein.

By proving a heretical thesis of an agent completely lacking nucleic acid, supporters of the thesis already confronted the next untouchable principle, namely that PrP^C and PrP^{Sc} differ only in their secondary and tertiary structure and not by alternative splicing [15] nor by chemical posttranslational modifications [154], leading to the so far unimaginable fact of a protein acquiring two possible secondary and tertiary structures, but with PrP^{Sc} working as template to support the probably energetic less efficient, synthesizing $t_{1/2}$ around 5 h for PrP^C but around 15 h for PrP^{Sc}, β-sheet dominated form, which in turn creates a protease resistance [22].

Although it is Prusiner who is known today as the founder of the protein-only hypothesis, there were two men preceding him with this novel idea. In 1967, John Stanley Griffith and Tikvah Alper, the former a mathematician, the latter a radiation biologist, published the thesis that proteins alone might be the causative agent of transmissible spongiform encephalopathies [3, 77].

1.1.3 Prion protein theory remains disputable

For his enduring work and tremendous findings, Stanley B. Prusiner was rewarded with the Nobel Prize in Physiology or Medicine in 1997, although the thesis of PrP^{Sc} being the solely pathogenic agent still remains questioned. There is data continuously being published suggesting that nucleic acids are involved in the pathogenesis of prion diseases. Heino Diringer, for example, sees a virus as the partner agent in which the virus is coated by PrP^{Sc} particles. It was in 1984 that he described Scrapie infected hamster as having a sustained viremia post infection [55], and in 1990 he explained that PrP^{Sc} was able to overcome species barriers in order to match viral patterns [56]. This was followed by a statement published in 1995, when he argued that the link between Scrapie and Creutzfeld-Jakob disease could be explained by the general rules of viral transmission [57]. Two years later he also managed to isolate a small amount of DNA out of brain matter from diseased animals, but was not able to further specify it [58]. In 2001, Diringer published his most recent postulation, where he argues the alternative thesis that a yet undiscovered virus-like agent may be the cause of transmissible spongiform encephalopathies.

However, the idea of a nucleic acid being an essential partner of Scrapie prion is supported by the emerging idea that RNA particles play a key role in the eruption of prion disease. It has been shown that RNA particles bind to PrP^C and stimulate its conversion to PrP^{Sc} *in vitro* [1, 52]. Additionally, an ambivalent interaction is described for DNA, where it was shown by Cordeiro et al. to catalyze conversion from an α-helical to a β-sheet structure on the one side, but, on the other, the binding of PrP^{Sc} with specific short DNA sequences prevents aggregation of the same [49].

Frank O. Bastian has challenged Prusiner since 1979 with his thesis that *Spiroplasma mirum* is the infectious agent in TSEs. It was then that he was first able to find *spiroplasma* like inclusions in biopsy material of a CJD patient using electron microscopy [16]. This finding was backed up shortly after in 1980 by Gray, who was also able to detect those *spiroplasma* like inclusions [76]. The definitive detection of *Spiroplasma*, however, was not until 2004, where Bastian was able to prove the presence of this bacterium in a high percentage of scrapie brains, CWD infected tissues and in CJD patients [18]. This was supplemented by the fact that an experimental GT-48 *Spiroplasma* infection in rodents caused a clinical and pathological picture remarkably similar to TSE. He accounted the lack of immune response in a body infected by bacteria to the high methylation rate of the *Spiroplasma*'s DNA making it invisible to toll receptors [17]. Indeed his thesis can be backed up by findings of other scientists like Forloni, who showed in 2002 that the prion protein infectivity is strongly affected by tetracyclines. He showed not only a decrease in PrP^{Sc} levels, but was also able to prevent hamsters scrapie in one third of the population [67]. This proved to be an interesting find because of Bastian's claim that *Spiroplasma* are resistant to every antibiotic product except tetracyclines [17]. As with Diringer, the argumentation for *Spiroplasma* also relies on the observed initial species barrier of PrP^{Sc}, which often is overcome in a very short time [160]. Bastian interprets this as a mutation and an adaption of *Spiroplasma* [17]. Additionally, he explains the report of chronic wasting disease (CWD) in deer being transmitted through contaminated grounds after a field was laid fallow for many years [185] to be caused by infectious bacterial reservoir [17]. However, recent studies also show that prion proteins bind to ground metals with a very high affinity [99], while also increasing their infectivity by a factor of a thousand, and show a durability under extreme conditions that enables a reservoir of persistent infectivity to last for years [227].

From these opposing argumentations it at least can be concluded, whether prion protein is the sole player in TSEs, or a virus, nucleic acids, *Spiroplasma* or others are essentially involved as well, that PrP^C plays a major role, and that the understanding of its function remains of tremendous importance.

1.2 The physiological function of PrP^C

1.2.1 Characterization of PrP^C

The prion protein is characterized by mainly two isoforms, PrP^C and PrP^{Sc}, with "C" standing for "Cellular" and "Sc" for "Scrapie", which is the infectious form. It is a glycoprotein which contains a phosphatidylinositol glycolipid, called a GPI anchor, responsible for attaching the protein to the outer plasma membrane and being able to be detached by phospholipase C [187]. The human prion protein is located on chromosome p20 and codes for 253 amino acids. PrP^C has a molecular weight of 35-36 kDa, one disulfide bond between the cysteine residues at 179 and 214, N-linked glycosylation sites at position 182 and 198, and a mainly α-helical structure in PrP^C (figure 1). As described later, the PrP^C has suspected ties to several cellular functions, all of which seeming to depend on the N-terminus, more precisely residues 23-31, with an amino acid sequence of KKRPKPGGW [197]. It is associated with almost every discussed function of PrP^C, especially with its biosynthetic pathway as a membrane or secreted protein, starting with its translation in the rough endoplasmic reticulum by its secretion through the Golgi apparatus, its cell surface expression followed by its clathrin dependent endocytic trafficking and degradation [201]. Most importantly, an extension of the above mentioned residues, from 23 to 90, form a second signal for transmembrane anchoring representing a proteinaceous raft targeting signal with the ectodomain of a GPI-anchored protein. Additionally it serves as a signal sequence, helping the PrP^C in its challenging mechanism of internalization. Since its outer membrane localization is in detergent insoluble lipid rafts, it would need a cytoplasmic domain to engage adapters to recruit them into clathrin coated pits, a domain PrP^C does not have. Therefore the N-terminal residues 27-107 guide the PrP^C from its normal lipid rafts to a lateral boarding detergent soluble spot where it can enter clathrin coated pits [197].

Besides its expression as a secreted membrane protein, it can also be found as a transmembrane and as a cytosolic isoform. There are actually two transmembrane forms, both having a conserved hydrophobic sequence which can span the lipid bilayer in either a C-terminal or N-terminal direction, therefore being called CtmPrP or NtmPrP, respectively. The expression of the CtmPrP also seems to correlate with Scrapie typical neurodegeneration as shown in recent data by Chakabarti [44]. The data for a cytoplasmic version, on the other hand, is more controversial, with recent studies suggesting that the observed cytoplasmic PrP is an artefact of trials with proteasome inhibitors, since proteasomes are normally responsible for degrading all cytoplasmic prion protein in an overexpressing status [61]. Moreover, cytoplasmic PrP seems to be strongly neurotoxic in cultured human cells and transgenic mice, showing severe ataxia with cerebellar degeneration and gliosis [122].

Introduction

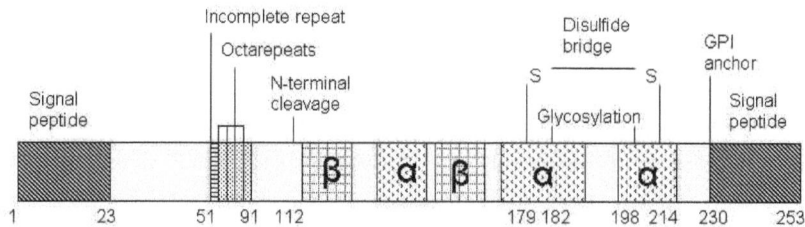

Figure 1: Schematic primary structure of human PrP^C

The N- and C-terminal signal peptides ranging from residues 1 to 23 and 231 to 253 are cleaved within the endoplasmic reticulum, while the GPI anchor is fixed on serine 230. Four Cu^{2+} can be bound at the octapeptide repeats from residues 51 to 91. Residues 182 and 198 are possible spots for N-linked glycolysation. The normal metabolic cleavage takes place at residue 112. A disulfide bridge is formed between cysteine 179 and 214. α, alpha-helix; β, beta sheet; GPI, glycosyl-phosphatidyl-inositol; S, sulfor.

Besides the cellular expression pattern, it is of equal importance how PrP^C is expressed in a more macroscopic view, especially where it concerns infectious routes. While almost all neurons express mRNA of PrP^C already during embryogenesis [124] only a specific collection actually expresses the protein on its surface, therefore suggesting a posttranscriptional control by differences in trafficking and/or degradation [65]. The highest levels of expression are observed in the so called hardwired neuroimmune network which integrates the body's immune defence and neuroendocrine systems under CNS control, including glial cells, small diameter nerves in the skin and lamina propria of the aerodigestive tract, sympathetic ganglia and nerves, dendritic cells, lymphocytes in skin, gut- and bronchus-associated lymphoid tissues, parasympathetic and enteric nervous system, peripheral axons and Schwann cells [66]. Furthermore PrP^C is involved in anterograde and retrograde axonal transport [138], and is concentrated in pre-synaptic terminals [13]. This includes the neuromuscular junction, where it seems to have an effect on afterhyperpolarization potentials [83] as well as in hippocampal cells [123].

1.2.2 PrP$^{0/0}$ – lack of phenotype

The first experiments done to further investigate the function of PrP^C were done in an attempt to delete the prnp gene and to observe the resulting phenotypical chnages. However, the first PrP-null mice in which only the coding regions were deleted (called Zurich I and Edinburgh mice) showed no distinctive phenotype compared to wildtype [36, 125]. A second PrP$^{0/0}$ line, called Nagasaki, showed severe ataxia and degeneration of purkinje cell, which was abolished by the reintroduction of *Prnp* [140, 169]. However, this was later proved to be due not to be the missing PrP^C, but instead

Introduction

to the different deletion technique, which caused the neighbouring Doppel protein (Dpl) to be regulated by the *Prnp* promoter, therefore causing an overexpression of Dpl [136].

A more detailed investigation of PrP^C deficient mice showed changes in the glutamatergic system and a preserved dopaminergic and adenosinergic system [48]. Furthermore, those animals showed an altered circadian rhythm similar to Fatal Familial Insomnia (FFI), suggesting a pathogenesis by loss of function [203]. An overexpression of PrP^C restored the physiologic status [64], while mRNA levels of PrP^C seemed to be circadian dependent [41]. Additional lack of prion protein causes an easy interruption of sleep, the mice presenting themselves as more wakeful [202].

1.2.3 PrP^C as an antiapoptotic agent

Prion protein has been proposed to interact with several enzymes (Table 2); one of the major fields that PrP^C relates to is the regulation of apoptotic mechanisms by members of the Bcl-2 protein family. BH3 triggers apoptosis by binding to pro-survival relatives while Bax (Bcl-2 associated protein X) and Bak (Bcl-2 antagonist killer 1) have a downstream role involving disruption of organellar membranes, mitochondrial translocation, cytochrome c release and induction of caspase activation. Additionally BH3 probably plays a stress sensor function and activates Bax and Bak, seen as a conformational change [206]. In primary neuronal cells and in human breast carcinoma cells (MCF-7), PrP^C prevents the initial conformational change of Bax, thereby blocking its apoptotic mechanisms while not influencing Bak and BH3 [165]. It was seen in a different study that the plasmid injection of fetal neuron cells not expressing PrP^C with Bax leads to an apoptosis rate of 90%, but, if Bax is co-injected with the PrP gene, the apoptosis rate declines to 10% [166]. Those results were also repeated in the model organism *Saccharomyces cerevisiae*, also known as baker's yeast. Although *S. cerevisiae* normally do not express endogenous Bcl-2 family or any caspases, if a Bcl-2 containing plasmid is injected in the yeast organism, the initial Bax events are similar to those in mammals. In a scenario of yeast being injected with Bcl-2 containing plasmids coupled to a galactose promoter once lacking and once supplemented with the PrP gene, proliferation is only seen in a galactose medium with *S. cerevisiae* being co-injected with PrP^C, while in a control series with a glucose medium no growth is seen at all. Additionally, these findings are connected to the secretory pathway, since PrP23-231, a cytosolic version, does not show a rescue activity. Furthermore, the charged region of residues 23-31 proves to be essential, while the octapeptid region does not influence the results [117], but does in human neurons [60] as well as in the deletion of the C-terminal GPI anchor [24], but resulting in the creation of amyloid plaques reminiscent of Alzheimer's disease [46]. PrP^C accumulates in Aβ-plaques most likely as a response to oxidative stress [130].

The above data was accidentally confirmed in investigations regarding TNFα resistance of different MCF-7 cell lines where a 17-fold overexpression of PrP^C is documented in those resistant to TNFα. This overexpression seems to alter cytochrome c release and nuclear condensation [53].

Completive to those observations, it was documented that Dpl (Doppel), a paralogue of PrP^C and proapoptotic in Prn-$p^{0/0}$ mice as well as in human neuroblastoma cells (N2a). are saved by overexpression of PrP^C [60, 158]. Experiments with Prn-$p^{0/0}$ mice started in 1992, but did not yield much information since those mice showed normal development and no deficits but were also resistant to PrP^{Sc} [36]. On the other hand, a mutation called PrPΔN which is the deletion of residues 32-121, presents with a Scrapie pattern and neuronal death of the infected mice 1-3 months after birth. This toxic effect is been reversed by a single copy of wtPrP [178], a result confirmed by an analogous experiment with Tg mice lacking residues 105-125 in which lifespan is elongated above one year by a five-fold overexpression of wtPrP [117].

1.2.4 Transmembranic signalling pathways

Although there is now accumulating data about the possibility of PrP^C acting in a neuroprotective way, i.e. in an antiapoptotic manner, it is questionable how the exact interaction takes places (Table 2). Because it resides in lipid rafts and is mainly endocytosed by a clathrin-dependent mechanism,, an adaptor protein is essential. Those include caveolin-1, which in turn activates signalling proteins like tyrosine-kinase-Fyn and –Src [200]. This endcytotic activation of Fyn makes it possible to activate NADPH oxidase and extracellular regulated kinases (ERKs) further downstream in neurons, which in turn have pro-survival effects [177].

Another well defined interaction occurs with STI1. In this case residues 113-128 of PrP^C bind to residues 230-245 of STI1, which in turn supposedly induces neuroprotective signals [233] by activating ERK and PKA pathways, which protect retinal explants from anisomycin induced apoptosis [47]. Furthermore PrP^C promotes neuritogenesis by modulating the interaction of astrocytes with neurons by STI-1 and laminin [118], which in turn requires the activation of the MAPK pathway in the neuronal cell [121]. However, the effect on proliferation and differentiation of PrP^C and STI1 is not only limited to neurons, but also extends to astrocytes itself where PrP^C and STI1 regulate survival and differentiation in a PKA and PKC dependent manner [7]. In turn, PrP^C influence in neuronal differentiation and proliferation was observed in adult stem cells from the subventricular zone with a so far undefined mechanism [188]. Pathways of neuritogenesis also appear to play a role in cerebral ischemic events. In comparison to Prn-$p^{0/0}$ mice, wtPrP mice are more capable in handling transient or permanent ischemia [219], which correlates with an upregulation of the PKB/PI-3 kinase, an enzyme that not only influcnes oxidative stress pathways, but also PKC and Src- and Fyn-kinases, which affect neuritic outgrowth as well [104]. Not to mention that the direct interactors NCAM and laminin are likewise major players in neuritogenesis, especially NCAM, which serves as an transmembrane adaptor to activate the pro-proliferative Fyn-kinase [175].

Tab. 2: Putative PrP^C interactors (Westergard et al. (2007) [222] and Linden et al. (2008) [119])
Grb2, growth factor receptor-bound 2; Pint-1, Prion protein interactor 1; TREK-1, two-pore potassium channel 1; NRAGE, neurotrophin receptor-interacting MAGE (melanoma antigen family) homologue; STI-1, stress inducible protein 1; Hsp60, heat shock protein 60 kDa; NCAM, neuronal cell adhesion molecule 1; GPI, glycosyl-phophatidyl-inositol; Bcl-2, B-cell lymphoma 2; ER, endoplasmic reticulum; PSD-95, post synaptic density 95; GASP, G associated sorting protein; 14-3-3, 14th fraction of bovine brain homogenate and were found on positions 3.3 of subsequent electrophoresis; CK2, casein kinase 2; Fyn, proto-oncogene tyrosine-protein kinase; ZAP-70, zeta-chain-associated protein kinase 70; PTPD1, protein tyrosine phosphatise; Fbx6, F box protein 6; Fbxo2, F box only protein 2; GFAP, glial fibrillary acidic protein; DNA, deoxyribonucleic acid; RNA, ribonucleic acid; hnRNP, heterogeneous nuclear ribonucleoproteins; Nrf, NF-E2-related factor; BiP, binding protein; GRP78, glucose regulated protein 78; APLP1, amyloid precursor like protein 1.

Candidate interactor	Candidate function	Localization
Grb2	Signal transduction (adaptor protein)	Cytoplasm
Pint1	Unknown	Cytoplasm
Synapsin 1b	Synaptic vesicle trafficking	Cytoplasm (vesicles)
TREK-1	Two-pore K$^+$ channel	Transmembrane
Tubulin	Microtuble subunit	Cytoplasm
NRAGE	Activator of apoptosis	Cytoplasm
Laminin receptor precursor	Extracellular matrix interactions	Cytoplasm
STI-1	Heat shock protein	Cytoplasm
Hsp60	Chaperone	Cytoplasm
NCAM	Cell adhesion	Transmembrane or GPI anchored

Bcl-2	Multi-domain antiapoptotic regulator	Cytoplasma, mitochondria, ER
Caveolin-1	Caveolar coat	Plasma membrane (hairpin loop)
PSD-95	Scaffolding protein	Transmembrane
GASP	G-Protein coupled receptor-associated sorting protein	Transmembrane
14-3-3	Scaffolding protein, cell signaling	Intracellular
CK2	Protein kinase	Intracellular
Fyn, ZAP-70	Protein tryrosine kinases	Membrane associated
PTPD1	Protein tyrosine phosphatase	Cytosolic
Aldolase C/zebrin II	Glycolytic pathway enzyme	Cytosolic
Fbx6/Fbxo2	Substrate recognition unit of ubiquitin ligase complex	Cytosolic
GFAP	Intermediate filament protein	Cytosolic
DNA	Nucleic acid	Nuclear
RNA	Nucleic acid	Nuclear / Cytosolic
hnRNP A2/B1	RNA-binding protein	Nuclear
Nrf2	Transcription factor	Nuclear
αB-crystallin	Stress-induced small hsp	Extracellular
BiP/Grp78	Endoplasmic reticulum chaperone	Endoplasmic
Laminin	Extracellular matrix component	Extracellular
β-Dystroglycan	Transmembrane protein	Transmembrane
APLP1	Amyloid precursor-like protein	Cytosolic
Heparin/heparin sulphate	Glycosaminoglycans	Extracellular

It is not just PrP^C which seems to be highly dependent on interacting proteins, but also a toxic version, PrP106-126, which has similar characteristics as PrP^{Sc}. In this case, toxicity is achieved by triggering a ROS overflow and over-activation of ERK/MAPK and SAPK consisting of p38 and JNK1/2. Those actions rely on cell surface expression of PrP^C and recruitment of a PrP^C-caveolin-Fyn signalling platform and NADPH oxidase activity. This provides evidence that PrP106-126 induced neuronal injury is caused by an amplification of PrP^C associated signalling responses, which promote an oxidative stressful environment [148]. The question of how this model can be applied to the relationship between PrP^{Sc} and PrP^C remains open.

1.2.5 Oxidative stress

The relationship between PrP^C and oxidative stress will account for most of the experiments and discussion shown later on, and a closer look at this relationship is necessary, as it has already been reviewed by Barry Halliwell [79]. Oxidative Stress describes a situation in which an organism is exposed to an environment filled with particles with a high reduction-oxidation (redox) potential. Those particles are called radicals or reactive oxygen species (ROS), although oxygen is not a radical requirement. Radicals or ROS, in turn, are any species capable of independent existence that contains one or more unpaired electrons. The most common radicals are formed by O_2 and its derivates, while another dangerous group is built up by transition metal ions like $Fe^{2+/3+}$ and $Cu^{2+/3+}$ of which it is known that copper is bound by prion protein (see 1.2.6). Further, these metals have the possibility to change between variable oxidation states, and therefore transfer single electrons which facilitates redox reactions. Thence uncaged transition metals are extremely dangerous. If a single electron is supplied to O_2, it enters one of the π antibonding oribitals to form an electron pair there, the product is a superoxide radical anion $O_2^{\cdot-}$ which actually is despite its name less reactive then O_2 itself. While $O_2^{\cdot-}$ are also a regular product of the respiratory chain. By adding another electron to the anion, it can react with $2H^+$ to form H_2O_2 a process which is catalyzed *in vivo* by superoxide dismutase (SOD) where a Cu/ZnSOD and a MnSOD can be distinguished. These metals in turn act as a reduction partner, but H_2O_2 itself is still a radical, which therefore is reduced by another four electrons and reacts with another $4H^+$ to form $2H_2O$, being catalyzed by catalase or glutathione.

Now if two radicals meet then a covalent bond is formed, but if a radical meets a non-radical, new radicals are created. One possibility is to add a radical to a DNA base, which would lead to a radical DNA adduct. This acts as a reduction agent like the later discussed Paraquat (PQ^{2+}), here PQ^{2+} becomes reduced to $PQ^{\cdot+}$ by cellular electron transport systems followed by $PQ^{\cdot+}$ reducing O_2 to $O_2^{\cdot-}$. Another possibility for a radical is to abstract a hydrogen atom from a C-H bond of fatty acid, leaving an unpaired electron on the carbon. This results in lipid hydroperoxide or even cyclic peroxides. This way a single initiation event has the potential to generate multiple peroxide molecules in a membrane by a chain reaction. The overall effects of this lipid peroxidation is a decrease in membrane fluidity, an easing of phospholipid exchange, an increased leakiness, a damage to membrane proteins and enzymes, receptors and ion channels which is done by amino acid oxidation. All this leads to a loss of membrane integrity and finally to cell death or apoptosis.

The connections between PrP^C and oxidative stress are diversified as well as disputable. One of the first approaches was done with rat phaechromocytoma PC12 cells in which was shown that, first, the toxic affect of the earlier described PrP106-126 depends on microglia to produce ROS. Auxiliary PC12 cells resistant to copper toxicity show increased levels of SOD and glutathione peroxidase [31]. In line with these results are findings in cell cultures lacking PrP^C expression undergoing cell death more rapidly when exposed to oxidative stress than wildtype cells. Additionally, PrP^C deficient cells show a lower level of Cu/ZnSOD and p53 but higher levels of the transcription factor NFκB [28, 33]. Consistent with these observations, wild type mice show a lower level of oxidative stress markers like lipid and protein peroxidation or ubiquitin-protein conjugates when compared to Prn-$p^{0/0}$ [228]. Very recent and reconfirmed data was presented from trials with hypoxia, which is supposed to cause part of its damage by elevating ROS levels. Whether transient ischemic or permanent, in living mice or in human hippocampal cell cultures, in all cases mRNA of PrP^C and its final expression are elevated or show a protective effect [129, 172, 186].

Thus the question rises of how this protective pattern of PrP^C is controlled and conducted. Not going into to much detail at this point, it can be reduced to two main ideas, one of PrP^C acting directly, by having a Cu/ZnSOD activity [27, 34] which is discussed very controversially [102], another by acting indirectly controlling enzymatic activities of proteins such as Cu/ZnSODs, e.g. Prn-$p^{0/0}$ seem to have their SOD activity being reduced to 10-50% of normal [30, 33, 107] as well as catalase and glutathione [223], but these findings heavily questioned [92, 216].

Although the relationship between prion protein and oxidative stress is highly disputable, it supposably also is the key to the function of PrP^C. Not just because other neurodegenerative disorders are at least partly defined by the level of neurons being exposed to oxidative stress, as it is observed in Alzheimer's disease, Parkinson's disease, ALS, Friedreich's ataxia or Huntington's disease (reviewed in [79]), but also because the discussed influences of PrP^C on antiapoptotic agents and transmembrane signalling pathways can be easily integrated.

1.2.6 The role of copper

For all the functions discussed previously, the copper ion Cu^{2+} is of great relevance. It is an accepted fact that PrP^C comprises four N-terminal histidine-containing octapeptide repeats (PHGGGWGQ), which are able to bind up to four Cu^{2+} [29, 95, 110, 192] in a pH dependent and negative cooperative pattern [217]. Besides those octarepeats, PrP^C has two additional binding sites at residues 96 and 111 which are normally occupied by Ni^{2+}, but can be replaced by Cu^{2+} [101].

The reasons for this or its consequences are not nearly as accepted. For example, a protease resistant prion form has been observed after binding Cu^{2+} [114], especially on residues 96 and 111 [100], but with a different characteristic than PrP^{Sc} [159]. The binding of Cu^{2+} also seems to stimulate endocytosis of PrP^C, which is achieved by a lateral movement of PrP^C out of the lipid raft into detergent soluble regions where clathrin-dependent endocytosis may happen [107, 201]. Since this action is most commonly seen in synapses, a role in the synaptic Cu^{2+} release is proposed [26], and also heavily opposed, by conflicting data [216].

Therefore, the role of copper in Prion protein remains debatable, but it is also obvious that the binding of Cu^{2+} is a cornerstone of the PrP^C function, making further research indispensable.

1.2.7 Non-neuronal function

PrP^C is not only an agent of neurons and glia cells, but is also found in the periphery. Prion protein is known to perform a regulator function in the immune system, and affects the ability of long-term hematopoietic stem cells to sustain self-renewal under stressful conditions [236]. Furthermore there is evidence of PrP^C interacting with the TCR complex and its downstream intracellular effectors like Src-family and non-receptor tyrosine kinase Fyn [128]. It has a positive effect on the differentiation and activation of dendritic cells [12], but a suppressive one on phagocytosis [51], while also enhancing leukocyte infiltration and peripheral inflammation processes [23].

However, besides its function in immune-modulation, one was also able to find increased expression rates of PrP^C in hereditary body mysositis and myopathy, polydermatomyositis and neurogenic muscle atrophy, although PrP^C shows a different glyocsylation profile and size than in brain matter [9, 234]. Elevated levels of PrP^C are also found in activated stellate liver cells [93] suggesting that prion protein is a reactive agent to stress in non-neuronal tissues.

1.3 Caenorhabditis elegans

1.3.1 Background of C. elegans

Caenorhabditis elegans, abbreviated *C. elegans*, is a free living nematode who lives in the soil across most temperate regions feeding on microorganisms. It requires only a humid environment, an ambient temperature, atmospheric oxygen and bacteria to feed on, requirements which make it easy and cheap to culture. It also always presents with the same amount of cells, enabling one to track each cell from the start as it further differentiates. Therefore, *C. elegans* was deliberately selected as a model system by Nobel Prize Winner Sydney Brenner in 1974, primarily because of its favourable characteristics regarding laboratory study and because of its glass like appearance, which makes it easy to investigate diverse processes, assuming that similar mechanisms would direct equivalent processes in all animal species [25]. Compared to the well established model system *Drosophila melanogaster*, it is superior not only because of its easiness in laboratory handling, but also regarding the similarity of its genome in relation to the human. Depending on which enzyme class you compare, the similarity ranges between 30 and 50%, with criteria for similarity requiring more than 90% of the protein's amino acid sequence to be identical [139].

The interest in these nematodes soared in response to the *C. elegans* genome project. It was the first multicellular organism for which the genome has been sequenced in 1998 [199]. Regarding research in the field of prion protein, *C. elegans* offers distinctive advantages. On the one hand, it does not express PrP^C as it has no Prnp gene. Further, *C. elegans* offers very well characterized (stress-) signalling pathways, therefore enabling an easy investigation of a possible exogenous PrP^C; in terms of gain of function. Most relevant is the transcription factor DAF-16 which is a member of the FoxO family. DAF-16/FoxO regulates numerous genes regarding, amongst others, antioxidants, chaperones, antimicrobials, apoptosis, growth, reproduction, development and metabolism [20]. DAF-16/FoxO, in its uncontrolled state, is located in the nucleus and activates gene expression. The DAF-2/IGF-1 signalling pathway, with three sub branches, is responsible for impeding the translocation of DAF-16/FoxO into the nucleus [84]. However, other signalling pathways promote translocation like SIR-2.1 [215]. The other important transcription factor regarding stress management besides DAF-16/FoxO is SKN-1/Nrf-2, which is controlled by p38/MAPK, however SKN-1/Nrf-2 also interacts with DAF-16/FoxO [97].

1.3.2 Anatomy of *C. elegans*

C. elegans appears in two sexes, male and hermaphrodite, the latter having both sperm and oocytes, enabling it to self-fertilize if there is no male available. The sperm of the male sperm is more fit than that of the hermaphrodite one. If cross-fertilization occurs males and hermaphrodites are produced in equal amounts, while self-fertilization produces only its own kind [87]. Both sexes have the same general anatomy (figure 2). On the genetic level, the male only has one sex chromosome (X0), while the hermaphrodite has two sex chromosomes (XX), but only has 959 somatic cells, including 302 nerve cells, while males have 1031 somatic cells, including 381 nerve cells. This excess of cells is due to its longer and more complex tail, which is necessary for the mating process. The mouth is at the tip of the head, and the anus of the hermaphrodite and cloaca of the male are ventral near the posterior of the worm. The gut, consisting of pharynx and intestine, runs straight from head to tail and can be visualized under the microscope because of its transparency, its very impressive pharyngeal pumping being responsible for transporting the bacterial food down the intestine. This is also the last vital sign of the worm to diminish [195]. The intestine is surrounded by the fluid-filled pseudocoelom containing four longitudinal bands of muscle cells, followed by a single-cell hypodermis, achieved by cell fusion, which in turn secretes a collagenous cuticle [2]. The sexual differences arise predominantly during post-embryonic development. In both sexes the gonad is a simple tubular structure with germ cells maturating along the tubular passage towards the exterior opening. Sperm cells are amoeboid like in all nematodes, while the uterus consists of two back reflexed tubes running anterior and posterior. The uterus is the localization where fertilization and part of embryogenesis take place [106, 194]. Most of the nerve cells are located around the circumpharyngeal nerve ring, the ventral nerve cord, the tail and differing sensory cells around the head. The nervous system is in charge to coordinate routine behavior and to respond to environmental stimuli. Most of the sensory neurons in the head and around the pharyngeal nerve ring have a chemosensory character. They comprise 40 neurons with dendrites facing toward the nose tip where they project to amphids which are bilaterally symmetrical sensilla and mediate non-volatile, chemical avoidance responses. There is at least one thermosensory neuron (AFD) in the head as well, and probably two special neurons (AQR, PQR) which report to the pseudocoelomic fluid, the equivalent of blood in mammals, acting as an osmotic regulator. Other sensory neurons are scattered throughout the body and tail and are mechanosensory [225]. In parallel to its sensory nerve system, it also has a somatic system to coordinate locomotion, a sinusoidal movement within a single dorsoventral plane. This movement is achieved by 95 body-wall muscles arranged in 4 longitudinal fibres with 24 cells each, with the exception of the left ventral which has 23 cells, with processes to the neuron serving as synapses instead of the other way around as in mammals. The nematode also commands several neural circuits, e.g. a avoidance reflex circuit or defecation motor circuit [180].

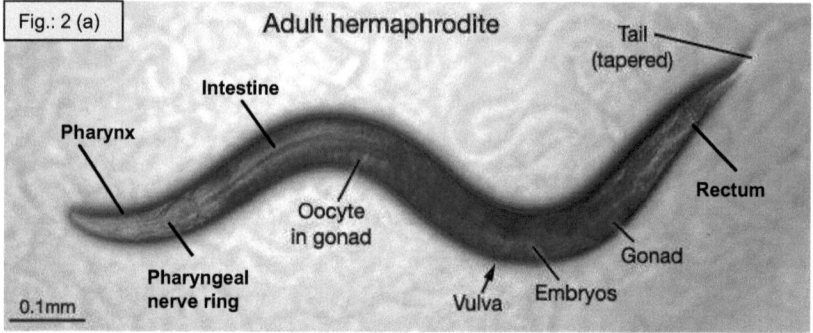

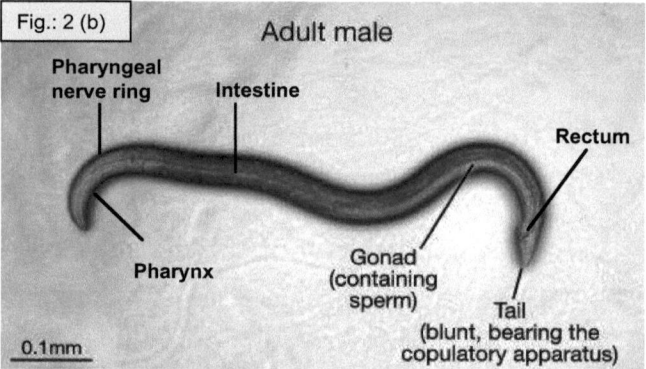

Figure 2:   Microscopic view of *C. elegans* (adapted from [90])
(a) Showing an adult hermaphrodite, all prominent characteristics are labelled; (b) Showing an adult male, all prominent characteristics are labelled.

1.3.3 Life cycle of *C. elegans*

The *C. elegans* has an average lifespan of around 17 days, depending on its environmental surroundings. Its developmental period from a laid egg to an adult worm is about three and a half days at 20 °C, while it is three days at 25 °C and six at 15 °C.

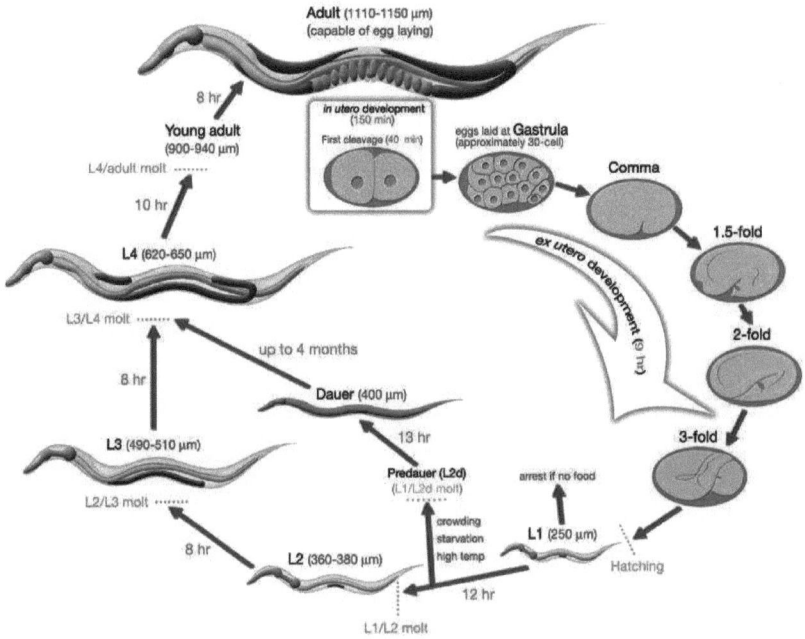

Figure 3: Stages of *C. elegans* development (obtained from [90])
The diagram shows important stages of *C. elegans* development. Starting at the top with the first cleavage in the hermaphrodite's uterus, five more embryogenic stages are seen characterized by the folds the worm appears under the microscope. After hatching four larval stages are stridden with two possibilities to adapt to food deprivation or population overgrowth, in L1 and L2/L3 stadium.

After hatching the worm undergoes four larval stages, L1 to L4 (figure 3), while L4 can be regarded as the adult worm, or young adult, since no further moults occur, and only a slight increase in size, to its maximum of about 1100 µm, remains in its development. If the worm suffers from adverse conditions like food deprivation, it is able to adapt to this situation by forming a dauer larval stage directly after the second moult instead of going into L3. This specialized form is thinner then the usual L3 stage and remains still, but moves faster in comparison when provoked. In this stadium it is viable for months and can moult to normal L4 when food becomes available. Another possibility is given during the L1 stadium, where, if there is a lack of food, the worm is able to arrest in this stadium and continue development as soon as the environment improves.

Embryogenesis takes around 12 h at 20 °C after fertilization and is divided into two phases, the intra- and extra-uterine phase. The initial intrauterine phase lasts around two and a half hours, while the extra-uterine phase lasts around 9 hours until the L1 worm hatches with an initial size of about 250 µm [87].

1.4   Objective of this work

As outlined previously. PrP^C still remains quite undefined regarding its physiologic function, the only certainty being its involvement in the infectious pathologic process of CJD and similar diseases by a shift in its secondary structure from a dominated α-helix pattern to a β-sheet pattern as it is seen in PrP^{Sc}. Its physiologic function remains open to debate, with many differing theories being discussed, and several different approaches being applied to solve this question. None of them, however, have provided specific hints for a superior model or testing approach.

Therefore, it is the objective of this scientific work to further investigate the physiologic function of PrP^C in the model organism *C. elegans*, which was used for the first time to express full length human PrP^C, following Kyung-Won Park and Liming Li first use in 2008 of *C. elegans* to express the pathogenic but artificial murine PrP(23-231) [145]. Since the theories about the prion protein function are wide spread, it was decided to constrain the research to the possible function of PrP^C influencing cellular management of oxidative stress. The main idea hereby is to compare the resistance of different genotypes in specific stress tests, which would allow one to infer the initial function of PrP^C.

2 Material and methods

2.1 Material

2.1.1 *C. elegans* strains

Strains were produced and obtained by Dr. rer. nat. Bettina Schulze and PD Dr. rer. nat Ekkehard Schulze, Bioinformatics and Molecular Genetics of Albert-Ludwigs-University in Freiburg, in cooperation with Prof. Dr. rer. nat. Oliver Hobert, Department of Biochemistry & Molecular Biophysics, Columbia University, New York, USA:

N2	*Wildtype*
GR1307	*DAF-16(mgDf50)I*
OH7600	*SOD-1(tm776)II*
EC410	*pha-1(e2123)III eeEx410[Psel-12::huPrPc(+) hmg-12::gfp pha-1(+)]*
EC411	*pha-1(e2123)III eeEx411[Psel-12::huPrPc(+) hmg-12::gfp pha-1(+)]*
EC418	*pha-1(e2123)III eeEx418[Psel-12::- hmg-12::gfp pha-1(+)]*
BR4955	*DAF-16(mgDf50)I pha-1(e2123)III eeEx410[Psel-12::huPrPc(+) hmg-12::gfp pha-1(+)]*
BR4905	*DAF-16(mgDf50)I pha-1(e2123)III eeEx411[Psel-12::huPrPc(+) hmg-12::gfp pha-1(+)]*
BR4907	*DAF-16(mgDf50)I pha-1(e2123)III eeEx418[Psel-12::- hmg-12::gfp pha-1(+)]* BR4992 *SOD-1(tm776)II pha-1(e2123)III eeEx410[Psel-12::huPrPc(+) hmg-12::gfp pha-1(+)]*
BR4966	*SOD-1(tm776)II pha-1(e2123) III eeEx411[Psel-12::huPrPc(+) hmg-12::gfp pha-1(+)]*
BR4993	*SOD-1(tm776)II pha-1(e2123)III eeEx418[Psel-12::huPrPc(+) hmg-12::gfp pha-1(+)]*
BR5306	*sod-4(gk101)III; pha-1(e2123)III eeEx411[Psel-12::huPrPc(+) hmg-12::gfp pha-1(+)]*

Material and methods

BR5307   sod-4(gk101)III;I eeEx418[Psel-12::- Phmg-12::gfp pha-1(+)]

BR5416   sod-4(gk101)III;I eeEx410[Psel-12::huPrPc(+) hmg-12::gfp pha-1(+)]

BR5124   =VC175 sod-4(gk101)III

BR5207   sod-5(tm1146)II; pha-1(e2123)III eeEx418[Psel-12::- hmg-12::gfp pha-1(+)]

BR5206   sod-5(tm1146)II; pha-1(e2123)III eeEx411[Psel-12::huPrPc(+) hmg-12::gfp pha-1(+)]

BR5205   sod-5(tm1146)II; pha-1(e2123)III eeEx410[Psel-12::huPrPc(+) hmg-12::gfp pha-1(+)]

BR5125   sod-5(tm1146)II

BR5044   pha-1(e2123)III eeEx(Psel-12::huPrPc(delta Okta) hmg-12::gfp pha-1(+))

To alleviate reading in the remaining text, appropriate names were used for above mentioned strains:

N2 – *wildtype*; GR1307 – *DAF-16 knock-out line*; OH7600 – *SOD-1 knock-out line*; EC410 – *PrP line 1*; EC411 – *PrP line 2*; EC418 – *plasmid line*; BR4955 – *DAF-16 knock-out PrP line 1*; BR4905 – *DAF-16 knock-out PrP line 2*; BR4907 – *DAF-16 knock-out plasmid line*; BR4992 – *SOD-1 knock-out PrP line 1*; BR4966 – *SOD-1 knock-out PrP line 2*; BR4993 – *SOD-1 knock-out plasmid line*; BR5306 – *SOD-4 knock-out PrP line 2*; BR5307 – *SOD-4 knock-out plasmid line*; BR5416 – *SOD-4 knock-out PrP line 1*; BR5124 – *SOD-4 knock-out line*; BR5207 – *SOD-5 knock-out plasmid line;* BR5206 – *SOD-5 knock-out PrP line 2*; BR5205 – *SOD-5 knock-out PrP line 1*; BR5125 – *SOD-5 knock-out line*; BR5044 – *Δ8*

2.1.2 Antibodies & cells

Antibody	Manufacturer
Anti PrP mAB 6H4	Prionics, Schlieren-Zürich, Switzerland
Anti PrP mAB 3F4	Covance, Princeton, USA
Peroxidase-conjugated Goat anti-Mouse IgG Polyclonal AB	Dianova, Hamburg

Cell	Manufacturer
Lymphocytes	Blutspendezentrale Ulm

2.1.3 Chemicals

Chemical	Manufacturer
Agar	AppliChem, Darmstadt
Agarose (4 %)	AppliChem, Darmstadt
Ampicillin	Ratiopharm, Ulm
Aprotinin	Roth, Karlsruhe
Bicinchoninic acid solution	Sigma-Aldrich, Taufkirchen
Bovine serum albumin	Paesel und Lorei, Duisburg
Buffer solution pH 4, 7, 9	AppliChem, Darmstadt
Calcium chloride dehydrate	Merck, Darmstadt
Cholesterol	Sigma-Aldrich, Taufkirchen
Coomassie	Serva, Heidelberg
Cupric I chloride	AppliChem, Darmstadt
Cupric sulphate	Sigma-Aldrich, Taufkirchen
Ethanol absolute	Sigma-Aldrich, Taufkirchen
ECL Plus system	Amersham Biosciences, Freiburg
5-Fluoro-2'deoxyuridine	Sigma-Aldrich, Taufkirchen
HEPES	AppliChem, Darmstadt
Iron II sulphate 7-hydrate	Roth, Karlsruhe
Magic Mark	Invitrogen, Karlsruhe
Magnsium sulphate heptahydrate	Merck, Darmstadt
Manganese Chloride	Sigma-Aldrich, Taufkirchen
Mercaptoethanol	Sigma-Aldrich, Taufkirchen
Methyl viologen dichloride hydrate	Sigma-Aldrich, Taufkirchen
Peroxidase anti-peroxidase	Sigma-Aldrich, Taufkirchen
Phosphate buffered saline	Biochrom, Berlin
PMSF	AppliChem, Darmstadt
Ponceau S	AppliChem, Darmstadt
Potassium phosphate	AppliChem, Darmstadt
Roti Load	Roth, Karlsruhe
SlowFade® Antifade Kit	Invitrogen, Karlsruhe
Sodium azide	AppliChem, Darmstadt
Sodium chloride	AppliChem, Darmstadt
Sodium duodecyl sulphate	Sigma-Aldrich, Taufkirchen

Material and methods

Sodium hydroxide	AppliChem, Darmstadt
Sodium hypochlorite solution	Hedinger, Stuttgart
SOD Buffer (10x)	Biomol, Ann Arbor, USA
SOD Standard	Biomol, Ann Arbor, USA
Tris Acetate EDTA buffer	Sigma-Aldrich, Taufkirchen
Tris buffered saline	Sigma-Aldrich, Taufkirchen
Trion X-100 (20%)	Biomol, Ann Arbor, USA
Trypton	AppliChem, Darmstadt
Roti-Load	Roth, Karlsruhe
Sodium deoxycholate	Sigma-Aldrich, Taufkirchen
WST-1 reagent	Biomol, Ann Arbor, USA
Xanthine oxidase	Biomol, Ann Arbor, USA
Xanthine solution (10x)	Biomol, Ann Arbor, USA
Yeast extract	AppliChem, Darmstadt
Zinc sulphate-7-hydrate	Riedel-deHaën, Seelze

2.1.4 Laboratory equipment

Equipment	**Manufacturer**
Axio Scope microscope	Zeiss, Oberkochen
Axiovert 200m microscope	Zeiss, Oberkochen
Biofuge fresco	Heraeus, Hanau
Biofuge pico	Heraeus, Hanau
Bottles (various sizes)	SIMAX, Boca Ration, Netherlands
Certomat H incubator	Sartorius Stedim Biotech, Aubagne Cedex, France
Electronic pipette	NUNC Wiesbaden
Electrophoresis power supply	Amersham Pharmacia Biotech, Munich
ELx 800 microplate reader	Bio-TEK Instruments, Bad Friedrichshall
Erlenmeyer flask	Duran, Wertheim/Main
Explorer balance	OHaus, Pine Brook, USA
Fridge (+4 °C)	Liebherr, Kirchdorf an der Iller
Freezer (-20 °C)	Liebherr, Kirchdorf an der Iller
Freezer (-80 °C)	Sanyo, Munich
GFL-3006 shaker	GFL, Burgwedel

Material and methods

Incubation closet	Binder, Tuttlingen
Microscope binocular (BMS)	Brunel microscopes LTD, Wiltshire, UK
Micro test tube rack	Brand, Wertheim
Microwave	Bosch, Gerlingen-Schillerhöhe
Mili-Q biocel A10 water filter station	Milipore, Billerica, USA
Mini Protean Tetra System electrophoresis	Bio Rad, Munich
MR 3001 magnetic stirrer	Heidolph, Schwabach
Multipipette	Corning, Corning, USA
PC	Dell, Round Rock, USA
pH electrode	Roth, Karlsruhe
Precision scales	Sartorius Stedim Biotech, Aubagne Cedex, France
RH basic 2 Mmgnetic stirrer	Janke & Kunkel IKA-Labortechnik, Staufen
TE 77 ECL Semi-dry transfer unit	Amersham Biosciences, Freiburg
Thermomixer comfort	Eppendorf, Hamburg
Typhoon 9400 fluorescence imager	Amersham Biosciences, Freiburg
VF2 vortex	Janke & Kunkel IKA-Labortechnik, Staufen

2.1.5 Consumption items

Item	Manufacturer
Combi tips	Eppendorf, Hamburg
Cover slip	Menzel-Gläser, Braunschweig
Delicate task wipes	Kimtech Science, Roswell, USA
Examination gloves	Semper Med, Vienna, Austria
Eyelashes	Own human resource, Ulm
Hybond-LFP	Amersham Biosciences, Freiburg
Micropipette (various sizes)	VWR, Darmstadt
Microscope slides Super Frost Plus	VWR, Darmstadt
Microtiter plates (96 wells)	Biomol, Ann Arbor, USA
Parafilm	Pechiney Plastic Packaging, Chicago, USA
Pasteur pipette	Brand, Wertheim
Petri dishes (3.5 cm; 6 cm; 9 cm)	Sarstedt, Nümbrecht

Material and methods

Pipet tips (various sizes)	VWR, Darmstadt
Safe seal tube (various sizes)	Sarstedt, Nümbrecht
Serological pipette	Sarstedt, Nümbrecht
Sterican	Braun, Melsungen
Tip Gilson/Eppendorf	Sarstedt, Nümbrecht
Tips Prot/Elec	Bio Rad, Munich
Toothpick	Fackelmann, Hersbruck
Top coat Rival de Loop	Rossmann, Burgwedel
Tubes (various sizes)	Sarstedt, Nümbrecht

2.2 Methods

2.2.1 Culturing and preparation of *C. elegans*

2.2.1.1 Preparation of NGM plates

In the laboratory *C. elegans* was maintained on Nematode Growth Medium (NGM) agar. It was aseptically poured into petri dishes of different sizes (35 mm, 60 mm and 90 mm) for different tasks [208]. The following protocol shows the standard procedure for NGM plates used for culturing worms. Aberrant methods for other tasks are explained in the following chapter.

Protocol – Preparation of NGM plates:

Equipment and reagents:
- Respective Petri plates
- 1.2 g NaCl
- 1.0 g Tryptone
- 6.8 g Agar
- 400 ml ddH$_2$O
- 400 µl MgSO$_4$ (1 M; autoclaved; stored at RT)
- 400 µl CaCl$_2$ (1 M; autoclaved; stored at RT)
- 400 µl Cholesterol solution (10 mg in 10 ml EtOH) stored at 4 °C
- 1x 400 ml screw-cap bottle
- Magnetic stirrer with hotplate
- Electronic pipette
- KPO$_4$ (pH 6.0) (1 M; autoclaved; stored at RT)

Procedure:

1. 1.2 g NaCl, 1.0 g Tryptone and 6.8 g Agar were added into a 400 ml bottle and dissolved in 400 ml ddH$_2$O, mixed with a magnetic stirrer and sterilized by autoclaving.
2. To get 1 M KPO$_4$ buffer: ddH$_2$O was added to 34.0 g KH$_2$PO$_4$ until the final volume of 250 ml 1 M KH$_2$PO$_4$ was obtained. Then ddH$_2$O was added to 45.6 g K$_2$HPO$_4$ till the final volume of 200 ml 1 M K$_2$HPO$_4$ is obtained. Afterwards K$_2$HPO$_4$ solution was added to KH$_2$PO$_4$ till a pH of 6.0. Following the potassium phosphate buffer was divided in 75 ml aliquots, autoclaved for 15 min liquid cycle and stored at RT.
3. After autoclaving, the mixture was kept at around 80 °C to avoid solidification for further procedure.
4. With the bottle standing on a magnetic stirrer with hotplate first 10 ml KPO$_4$ (ph 6.0), second 400 µl MgSO$_4$ (1 M) and 400 µl CaCl$_2$ (1M), third 400 µl Cholesterol solution were added while if possible working at a flow hood to avoid contamination.

5. Using an electronic pipette specific amounts of NGM were added to the Petri dishes: Amounts as follows:
    - 90 mm Petri plates: 20.0 ml NGM added
    - 60 mm Petri plates: 7.0 ml NGM added
    - 35 mm Petri plates: 3.5 ml NGM added
6. NGM plates were left overnight at room temperature to let the NGM cool down and to get rid of excess moisture.
7. Afterwards they were stored at 8 °C and used if needed. They remained usable for up to 4 weeks.

2.2.1.2 Preparation of growth media

During the whole research project *C. elegans* was maintained monoxenically, meaning *E. coli* strain OP 50 served as a single food source [25]. To do it axenically [208] is difficult and the growth of the animals would have been very slow. *E. coli* OP 50 was placed on NGM plates which limits growth of *E. coli* OP 50 as an uracil auxotroph. Limitation of bacterial growth is desirable for better observation and mating of the worms.

Protocol – Preparation of *E. coli* OP 50:

Equipment and reagents:

- 3 g Trypton
- 1.5 g NaCl
- 300 ml ddH$_2$O
- 1x 400 ml screw-cap bottle
- 6x 100ml screw-cap bottles
- 1x 500ml Erlenmeyer flask

- Magnetic stirrer
- *E. coli* OP 50
- Multitip Pipet
- Individual formed Pasteur pipet
- Shaking incubator
- Respective NGM plates

Procedure:

1. Making B-Broth: 3 g Trypton and 1.5 g NaCl were dissolved with 300 ml ddH$_2$O in a 400 ml bottle and mixed with a magnet stirrer, split up afterwards into 6 portions à 50 ml in 100 ml bottles and sterilized by autoclaving.
2. 50 ml of sterilized B-Broth were poured into a 500 ml flask. A piece of OP 50 stock, stored at -80 °C, was scraped of, and added to the above. The flask was covered again with the aluminium foil used for autoclaving.

3. Overnight the Erlenmeyer flask with ingredients was incubated at 37 °C at 220 rpm. If the colour of the solution had not changed from diaphanous to murk, it was incubated for another 24 h.
4. Using a multitip pipet the bacterial fluid was added to NGM plates as follows, if possible a Laboratory Bench was used to avoid contamination:
   - 90 mm NGM plates for worm culturing: 1000 µl dispensed each
   - 90 mm NGM plates for Paraquat stressing: 200 µl dispensed each
   - 60 mm NGM plates, all kinds: 200 µl dispensed each
   - 35 mm NGM plates for worm culturing: 50 µl dispensed each
   - 35 mm NGM plates for stressing, all kinds: 25 µl dispensed each
5. An individual formed Pasteur pipet was taken to streak out the bacterial fluid on the NGM plate, but the outer frame of the plate has been left out to prevent worms from curling up the edge.
6. Plates were left overnight at room temperature to let the fluid dry and bacteria grow. Afterwards they were stored at 8 °C. They remained usable for 2-3 weeks.

2.2.1.3 C. elegans in RNAi

For investigating the influence of the SKN-1/Nrf-2 stressway, it was chosen to inhibit the enzymatic function by blocking its protein translation using specific RNAi which in turn was produced by a specific *E. coli* strain. Its selection was connected to a broad antibiotic resistance.

To culture this *E. coli* strain on NGM plates, the procedure under 2.2.1.1 was supplemented by adding 400 µl of 1mM IPTG per 400 ml NGM as well as 112.5 µl of ampicillin with a stock concentration of 0.2 g/ml in step 3. In addition 100 ml of autoclaved B-Broth were supplemented by 25 µl of ampicillin using the same stock as above, as well as by 120 µl tetracycline with a stock concentration of 10 mg/ml. At no time did temperature rise over 50 °C. All other steps of preparation were identical to 2.2.1.2

The embryo test was done to determine the success rate of SKN-1/Nrf-2 RNA translation. SKN-1/Nrf-2 is an essential enzyme for embryogenesis, and therefore a lack of such would result in unhatchable eggs. To quantify the inhibition, L1 larvae were placed on those specific RNAi NGM plates, after 36 h the now adult worms were removed and the eggs counted. After another 8 h the hatched animals were counted in relation to the total egg number. A rate of unhatched eggs > 50% was regarded as successful inhibition.

2.2.1.4 *C. elegans* on NGM plates

Transparent *C. elegans* were visualized using a dissecting stereomicroscope equipped with a transmitted light source (Microscope binocular (BMS)) and objectives ranging from 0.7 to 4.5. Several methods were used to transfer worms from one plate to another.

If a whole bulk of worms needed to be transferred, a chunk of agar, around 1 x 1 cm, was cut out of the old plate with a 70% ethanol sterilized scalpel, transferred to a fresh seeded NGM plate and laid on top. This way a heterogeneous mass of worms, as well as those burrowed in the agar, were able to crawl out, spread and mate again. This method was used only for keeping worm stocks alive or to obtain a broad load of worms for frozen worm stocks or a heap of egg-loaded worms for further experiments. Advantages for this method included not being forced to work with a microscope, as well as the ability to transfer worms quickly, but it did not allow one to select the worms being transferred

In order to transfer many selected worms at once, a 2.5 cm piece of 32-gauge platinum wire was mounted to the tip of a Pasteur pipet. The end of the wire was flattened with a hammer and filed with an emery cloth to remove sharp edges to avoid the killing of worms and to avoid holes in the agar. One advantage of using platinum wire was quick heating and cooling. This way it could be sterilized easily by holding it over a flame after several picks or even after every pick. A disadvantage is the danger of damaging the agar or the worm and the amount of practices required to use it safely. To collect many worms at once, the wire was gently drawn over the agar with the flat side facing the agar, and surveying it through the dissecting microscope. The platinum wire was also used for picking single worms from one destination to the other. In this case a drop of at least two days old *E. coli* OP 50 was first collected on the tip of the wire before touching the top of the chosen worm. To release the worms onto a fresh plate, the wire had to be lowered slowly until it gently touched the surface of the agar, and was held there to allow the worms to crawl off the picker. The platinum wire was mostly used to transfer an entire load of young egg loaded worms to fresh plates for further experiments.

Another method for selective picking was to use a human eyelash mounted on the tip of a toothpick by fast hardening glue. This way even small single L1 worms could be hooked on the eyelash, transferred to another plate and fluffed off. Once a while, or, if necessary even after every pick, the picker was sterilized by 70% ethanol. This method was used to transfer specific worms in several procedures.

Frequency of transferring depended on further intentions. To receive cultures with animals at every stage, worms were transferred every 2-3 days. To keep a stock alive, transferring every 2-3 weeks was enough, but this also depended on the temperature, since worms stored at 25 °C grow 2.1 times faster then worms stored at 16°C [191]. As discussed later, some experiments forced transferring even after a few hours. Petri plates were always labelled by strain name and date for identification, and the cover was removed as little as possible to avoid any contamination.

Once *C. elegans* were transferred on seeded NGM plates, and were stored in sterilized cardboard boxes in an incubator at 25 °C with circulating air to keep humidity low. The temperature was chosen in respect to the *pha-1* gene located on the injected plasmid, which served as a selector for transgenic worms, allowing to mate and grow only those worms which were in possession of the plasmid *pha-1* gene, while the chromosomal *pha-1* gene was deleted.

2.2.1.5 Contamination and bleaching

Occasionally, NGM plates containing *C. elegans* became contaminated with mould, yeast or bacteria. This contamination normally does not harm the worm directly but it can influence biochemical pathways of the worm concerning calorie restriction, which would have had influences on several experiments [89]. Therefore, plates were cleaned as much as possible.

To get rid of contamination, a 1:1 mixture of 1 M NaOH and 12 % NaOCl, which resembles household bleach, was set up [193]. The mixture was made fresh when needed because of the tendency of the ingredients to react with each other. Also, NaOCl was stored in the dark at 8 °C to avoid self reaction by UV light. A 50 µl drop of the mixture was then placed on the edge of a clean 60 mm NGM plate seeded with *E. coli* OP 50. With the platinum wire pick several egg filled hermaphrodites were picked from the contaminated plate and placed into the bleaching drop. The worms ceased living immediately and their structure became dissolved, leaving only the eggs which were resistant to the bleach mixture because of their chitin layer. When the embryos hatched, the bleach was soaked into the agar and therefore could not cause any harm. But to make sure that all stress pathways of *C. elegans* were at a natural level and not increased by some of the remaining bleach, worms were cultured for another two generations using a new plate for each generation.

2.2.1.6 Synchronized cultures

For several experiments it was necessary to work with staged animals. The most common way is by working with liquid cultures, mass bleaching and seeding the retained eggs on fresh 90 mm NGM plates [87]. Because of the problems establishing this method and because of the amount of material and time that were needed, the possibility of influences on several stress pathways by remaining bleach could not be excluded. Therefore, a more uncommon but simple way was used as described previously [198].

Depending on the amount of staged animals needed, either 20-30 egg-filled hermaphrodites were placed on fresh 60 mm *E. coli* OP 50 seeded NGM plates or 150-200 on 90 mm plates for 1 h to let them lay their eggs either by using the toothpick or the platinum wire system, depending on the plates the worms were taken from. Afterwards, the adult worms were removed again. Nine h after egg laying the first embryos hatched, creating a population synchronized within a 1 h time span, which had no impact considering only adult worms were needed and a total lifespan of *C. elegans* of about 20 days neglecting the prior 1 h time difference. Worms were always stored at 25 °C. After around 46 h the synchronous population reached young adult stage and was ready for further investigation.

2.2.1.7 Frozen *C. elegans* stocks

To maintain different *C. elegans* strains at the same time it was necessary to store strains which were not needed for a period of time in form of Aliquots at a -80 °C freezer [191]. If *C. elegans* is frozen only L1-L2 stage animals are able to recover. Therefore, plates with starved animals were used, delivering the highest amount of L1 dauer larvae.

Protocol – Freezing *C. elegans*

Equipment and reagents:

- 3x Worm covered 90mm NGM plates
- 10x 1.5 ml Eppendorf tubes
- 1x Petri plate
- Microcentrifuge
- -80 °C freezer
- S buffer + 30% glycerol (v/v). Sterilized by autoclaving

- S buffer: 129 ml 0.05 M K_2HPO_4, 871 ml 0.05 M KH_2PO_4, 5.85 g NaCl. Sterilized by autoclaving
- Single use pipets
- Styrofoam box with holding slots
- 20 cm x 30 cm Styrofoam box filled with ice

Procedure freezing:

1. 3x 90 mm NGM plates covered with *C. elegans* were washed with around 4 ml S buffer using a single use pipet as through the whole protocol. The same 4 ml were used for all three plates. The 4 ml of S buffer worm solution were pipeted into 6x 1.5 ml Eppendorf tubes with around 660 µl each.
2. Eppendorf tubes containing worm solution was centrifuged for 5 min at 400 x g at 4 °C.
3. Afterwards the supernatant was aspirated and the pellet of worms was left over. The pellet was diluted again in 1 ml S buffer each.
4. Step 2-3 was repeated twice. After the 3rd time only three pellets were diluted again in 500 µl S buffer and transfused each to a tube without a diluted pellet.

5. Step 2
6. After aspirating the supernatant of the three left over Eppendorf tubes only two pellets were diluted again in 500 µl S buffer and transfused to the remaining tube.
7. Step 2
8. Supernatant was aspirated again and the pellet was dissolved again in 500 µl S buffer. The solution was then transferred to a Petri plate lying on ice.
9. The same amount of ice-cold 30% glycerol S buffer mix was then added to the cooled Petri plate containing the worm solution.
10. After mixing worm suspension and freezing solution gently for 2-3 seconds, the solution was then transferred to five already labelled 1.5 ml Eppendorf tubes with 200 µl each. The tubes were sorted into a Styrofoam box with holding slots and quickly moved to a -80 °C freezer. Step 10 was done as fast as possible to avoid *C. elegans* swallowing glycerol which would have killed them.
11. After 24 h one stock was unfrozen again to check the quality of the stock, the remaining were placed in a cryocarton for final storing.
12. To unfreeze the stock, the Eppendorf tube was warmed at 37 °C just enough so that the solution could be aspirated. It was then pipeted to the edge of a 90 mm *E. coli* OP 50 seeded NGM plate while leaving it uncovered to enable the solution to dry faster. Surviving worms then crawled onto the *E. coli* lawn.

2.2.2 Lifespan determination

2.2.2.1 Lifespan without 5-fluoro-2'-deoxyuridine

For all lifespan measurements, synchronous populations of nematodes at the young adult stage were reared as described under 2.2.1.6. For lifespan analysis, 20 young adult staged nematodes were each placed on 35 mm NGM plates with an overall amount of 100-200 nematodes for each strain. Placing time was recorded as t = 0. During the brood period, lasting about 5-6 days, adult nematodes were transferred to new plates every 24 hours. Following the brood period, adult animals were moved to new plates at eight day intervals to avoid food competition and possible starvation. Animals were judged as dead, counted and removed from the plate when they ceased pharyngeal pumping and did not respond to prodding with a platinum wire. The occasional animal that was lost due to crawling off the plate or desiccation on the sides of the plate was censored and excluded from analysis [54]. Contaminated plates were also excluded of the analysis. *C. elegans* were also kept at 25 °C at all times.

2.2.2.2 Lifespan with 5-fluoro-2'-deoxyuridine

For saving of labour and handling of bigger amounts of nematode strains, lifespan was determined using 5-fluoro-2'-deoxyuridine (FDUR) to suppress the production of their progenies [68] working as a nucleotide analogues. Lifespan results of wildtype (N2), PrP line 1 (EC410) and 2 (EC411), as well as plasmid line (EC418) were compared with results of the previous lifespan determination method indicating no differences and therefore no relevant influence on this testing. Plates containing 40 µM FDUR were produced by adding a hundredth of the total NGM volume of a 4 mM FDUR Stock solution to the NGM following autoclaving and after adding all the other ingredients written under chapter 2.2.1.1 Step 3. Nematodes were reared for all lifespan measurements as written under 2.2.1.6. Young adult staged worms were then transferred to FDUR NGM plates. After 24 h they were transferred on fresh FDUR NGM plates because of nematodes laying eggs already bred before FDUR supplementation. Following this period, nematodes were transferred to fresh FDUR NGM plates every eight days to avoid starvation and food competition. Worms were examined daily, and dead worms were removed to count. Worms dead by desiccation at the walls of plates were excluded from analysis. Nematodes on plates contaminated by other microorganisms were also excluded from analysis. *C. elegans* were again kept at 25 °C at all times.

2.2.3 Stress assays

2.2.3.1 Cu^{2+} induced toxicity

To find a way for stressing *C. elegans* with Cu^{2+} ions as a member of the heavy metal family and its toxic potential as an oxidative agent [98], it was not possible to rely on previous publications and descriptions because of broad varying data and information regarding this method. Therefore, the method and the right Cu^{2+} concentration had to be determined in preceding experiments. For easier comparison of the data of the different experiments, it was decided to continue testing nematodes on NGM plates [214] rather then in liquid cultures [14] as well as to test the overall lifespan instead of testing embryogenesis or larval development. A first test setup included 20 young adult staged worms each on five 35 mm Cu^{2+} FDUR NGM plates per concentration containing $CuSO_4$ in concentrations of 0, 0.5, 0.75, 1.0, 2.0 mM. $CuSO_4$ was added out of a 100 mM Stock solution to the NGM following autoclaving and after adding all the other ingredients written under chapter 2.2.1.1 Step 3, as well as adding FDUR as written in the previous chapter. Afterwards nematodes were checked every 12 h looking for any abnormalities regarding egg laying, larval development and fitness, showing that a concentration between 0.5 and 1.0 mM $CuSO_4$ probably result in the best analyzable data. Therefore, a final Cu^{2+} stress concentration of 0.8 mM $CuSO_4$ was chosen.

For Cu^{2+} stress testing 150 young adult staged nematodes were placed on ten 35 mm Cu^{2+} FDUR NGM plates containing 0.8 mM $CuSO_4$ and 40 µM FDUR. Plates were examined every 12 h for dead worms which was tested by touching their heads with a platinum wire to see if pharyngeal pumping ceased. Dead worms were removed and counted. Worms dead by desiccation at the walls of the plates or worms on plates contaminated by other microorganisms were excluded from analysis. *C. elegans* were again kept at 25 °C at all times. The overall time span lasting for about 9 days.

2.2.3.2 Paraquat induced oxidative stress

To investigate the influence of N,N'-Dimethyl-4,4'-bipyridinium dichloride commonly known as Paraquat, a producer of superoxide anions, on *C. elegans*, a comparable method to the other stress assays was chosen [11]. At this point it has to be told that Paraquat is a very toxic agent therefore working with Paraquat required the standard laboratory protection of glove, goggles and coat, wearing a mask and special attention to handling. Disposal of hazardous waste was coordinated with the responsible waste management of the laboratory.

Paraquat was obtained as a powder in darkened 1 g bottles. Three g of Paraquat were prepared at one occasion to receive 100 mM Paraquat FDUR NGM plates. Therefore, the protocol in chapter 2.2.1.1 was changed as follows:

1. 0.351 g NaCl, 0.296 g Trypton and 1.989 g Agar were added into a 400 ml bottle and dissolved in 80 ml ddH_2O, mixed with a magnetic stirrer and sterilized by autoclaving.
2. After autoclaving the mixture has been kept at around 80 °C to avoid solidification for further procedure.
3. With the bottle standing on a heating magnetic stirrer first 2.93 ml KPO_4 (pH 6.0), second 117 µl $MgSO_4$ (1 M) and 117 µl $CaCl_2$ (1M), third 117 µl Cholesterol and fourth 1.17 ml of 4 mM FDUR Stock were added while always working under a laboratory bench if not stated otherwise.
4. One Paraquat bottle was opened and the content was dissolved in 37 ml ddH_2O while shaking it carefully. The solution was then transferred to the second bottle until the contents were dissolved in the same way. Procedure was repeated with the third bottle. Afterwards the Paraquat solution was added to the prepared NGM solution.
5. Using a peristaltic pump, specific amounts of the Paraquat NGM were added to the Petri dishes: Amounts as follows:
    - 35 mm Petri dishes: 3.5 ml Paraquat NGM added
    - 90 mm Petri dishes: 7.0 ml Paraquat NGM added

6. Paraquat NGM plates were left overnight at room temperature to let the NGM cool down and to get rid of excess moisture.
7. Afterwards they were stored at 8 °C and used if needed. They remained usable for up to 1 week.

For the Paraquat stress assay young adult staged nematodes were placed onto 35 mm Paraquat FDUR NGM plates and were checked for body movement by poking them with a platinum wire every 1-2 h. Dead worms were removed and counted. If the body movement dropped from "regular" to "almost ceased" in a 2 h interval then the worm was counted dead as well because of the point of death being closer to the present interval then to the upcoming one. Before being able to make such decisions about point of death, the dying behavior was previously studied in several test runs. Plates were kept at 25 °C at all times. The overall time span lasting for about 24 h.

For the SOD Assay (2.2.4) a synchronized culture was washed off a 90 mm dish and pipetted in 2 ml Eppendorf tubes, centrifuged at 400 x g for 5 min and the supernatant was aspirated afterwards. The worm pellet was resolved in 500 µl ddH$_2$O and then transferred on 90 mm Paraquat NGM dishes. Worms were kept on those dishes for 2 h at 25 °C until they were washed off again followed by a cleaning process, i.e. centrifuging, supernatant aspiration and resolving three times. Thereafter they were processed as described in 2.2.4.

2.2.3.3 Paraquat following previous Cu^{2+} treatment

To determine the influence of Cu^{2+} on oxidative stress resistance in *C. elegans*, the methods under 2.2.3.1 and 2.2.3.2 were combined. Dishes were prepared as described in those previous chapters, the only difference being in the use of 0.2 mM of Cu^{2+} as a final concentration in 60 mm NGM plates instead of 0.8 mM in 35 mm plates as described earlier. As well as omitting FDUR in the Cu2+ dishes. The Cu^{2+} concentration of 0.2 mM was chosen because it was the highest possible concentration where nematodes could still perform normal reproduction and development as obtained in a self ran trial.

From well crowded plates containing a large amount of young adults, a chunk of agar was cut out as described in 2.2.1.4 for each tested line and placed on a 0.2 mM Cu^{2+} plate. After 4 days, a chunk was cut out of the crowded Cu^{2+} plates and placed on a fresh 0.2 mM Cu^{2+} plate. This step was repeated another three times obtaining the 4th generation of young nematodes living on Cu^{2+} containing NGM plates. Then 20 young pregnant adults were placed for each line on fresh Cu^{2+} plates and removed after 1 h. After 46 h, a synchronized culture for each line was obtained and tested on Paraquat as described in 2.2.3.2. A control population was always tested in parallel with no Cu^{2+} background to make results comparable with previous findings.

2.2.3.4 Heat stress

To observe the behavior of *C. elegans* in handling increased heat, a quite common and established way was chosen [11]. After obtaining synchronous cultures as described in 2.2.1.6 for each tested line, 20 young adult staged worms were placed on 35 mm plates, incubated at 36 °C ± 0.4 °C and scored every one or two hours as dead or alive by checking for pharyngeal pumping by touching them with a platinum wire. The overall time span lasted for about 12 h.

2.2.3.5 Hydrogen peroxide induced toxicity

Hydrogen peroxide (H_2O_2), a cytotoxic agent, acting as an oxidative cellular stressor requiring breakdown by catalase like enzymes, was used for further investigations [138]. Published protocols [11] [96] were not realizable.

Two more or less satisfying protocols were obtained on the authors' own initiative. In the first version, 2.0 mM H_2O_2 35 mm dishes were manufactured by adding 30% H_2O_2 solutions to liquid NGM before pipetting it to 35 mm plates. 20 Young adult staged nematodes were then placed on those H_2O_2 plates for 45 min at 25 °C. Afterwards they were removed and placed on normal 35 mm FDUR plates. Plates were examined for dead worms every hour for the first 12 h, followed by every 4 h for another 24 h and finally every 24 h. Nematodes were stored at 25 °C at all times.

In the second version, 1.7 mM H_2O_2 35 mm dishes were manufactured by adding 30% H_2O_2 solutions to liquid NGM before pipetting it to 35 mm plates. 20 Young adult staged nematodes were then placed on those H_2O_2 plates and examined for dead nematodes every 24 h. Worms were stored at 25 °C at all times.

2.2.4 SOD assay

SOD Assay was performed using a Superoxide Dismutase Activity Kit provided by Biomol GmbH, and the protocol given by the manufacturer for preanalytical preparation of various samples was adapted to *C. elegans*.

Protocol – SOD Assay in *C. elegans*:

Equipment and reagents:
- Clear 8x12 microtiter plates uncoated
- SOD Standard
- 10x SOD buffer
- Xanthine Oxidase
- 10x Xanthine solution
- 20% Triton X-100
- WST-1 Reagent
- 10x PBS
- 0.154 M KCN
- chloroform/ethanol (37.5/62.5 (v/v))

- ddH$_2$O
- Protease inhibitors (PMSF, Aprotinin)
- C. elegans preparations
- Eppendorf tubes 0.5, 1.5 and 2.0 ml
- 15 falcon tubes
- Precision pipets ranging 10 to 1000 µl
- Multichannel pipets
- Centrifuge (cooled to 4 °C)
- Ice
- ELISA reader plus software

Procedure worm preparation:

1. Synchronous populations of different *C. elegans* strains were obtained as described in 2.2.1.6. Three or four crowded 90 mm plates with staged young adults were then washed of with ddH$_2$O as described in 2.2.1.7 under step 1 – 7, except for the use of ddH$_2$O instead of S buffer and 2 ml microtubes instead of 1.5 ml. The remaining pellet was then stored at -80 °C for 24 h. The timeframe was chosen only for matters of cmparison.
2. Pellets were thawed again keeping them at around 4 °C at all times by working on ice. The pellets were span down for 5 min at 9450 x g at 4 °C. The supernatant was removed and discarded.
3. The pellet was then resolved again in 4x volume shares of 1x PBS containing 0.2 M PMSF and 1 µg/ml Aprotinin.
4. Afterwards the solution was homogenized by an ultrasound rod using 4 repeats with a cycle of 9 and duration of 10 s. The 2.0 ml Eppendorf tubes were kept on ice the entire time, as ultrasound threatened to cause severe warming. Care was taken that the ultrasound rod not touch the Eppendorf, as this would have caused ebullition of the solution.
5. Previously prepared 5x Cell extraction buffer (5 ml of 10x SOD buffer, 1.0 ml of 20% Triton X-100, 0.2 M PMSF and 4.0 ml of ddH$_2$O) was added to the homogenate and vortexed extensive for 40 s.
6. The homogenized samples were then incubated on ice for 30 min and vortexed periodically.
7. Following incubation the lysate was centrifuged at 9450 g for 10 min at 4 °C. Afterwards the supernatant was pipeted to fresh 1.5 ml Eppendorf tubes, using 5 tubes for each line containing about 200 – 300 µl of lysate each depending on the pellet volume of worms used from the beginning. Around 50 µl from each strain were kept for determining protein concentration (see 2.2.5)
8. Aliquots were then immediately frozen in liquid N$_2$ and stored at -80 °C for further use. The following day the assay was continued.

Procedure SOD Assay:

Material and methods

1. 1x Xanthine solution was prepared by diluting 10x Xanthine solution with 1x SOD buffer by factor 1:10. 1x SOD buffer itself was obtained by diluting 10x SOD buffer with ddH$_2$O. The total volume was computed by "number of wells being used" times 25 µl. Final solution was then stored on ice

2. Master Mix was prepared by mixing 0.1 otv of 10x SOD buffer with 0.033 otv of WST-1 Reagent with 0.033 otv of Xanthine Oxidase with 0.833 of ddH$_2$O. The total volume was computed by "number of wells being used" times 150 µl. The final solution was stored on ice.

3. For differentiation of SOD-1 to SOD-5 for each sample three specific stocks of 200 µl volume each were prepared. To inhibit the activity of Cu/ZnSODs, that were SOD-1, -4 and -5 one stock was mixed with 3.91 µl of 0.154 M KCN to get a final concentration of 2 mM CN$^-$, thereby inhibiting over 90% of Cu/ZnSOD activity by forming a complex with Cu^{2+} of the mentioned SOD. To get rid of MnSOD activity, that were SOD-2 and -3, 320 µl of ice-cold chloroform/ethanol (37.5/62.5 (v/v)) were added to another stock, vortexed and centrifuged at 2500 g for 10 min. The supernatant was removed and used for the assay. The third stock was kept unchanged. Stocks were kept on ice at all times.

4. Depending on the results of the protein concentration determination (2.2.5), four gradient sample dilutions in a range from 5 to 0.5 µg/µl were obtained using an undiluted solution for the highest concentration. The other three dilutions were obtained by mixing a previous calculated amount of sample solution with 1x SOD buffer in a 0.5 ml micro tube so that an overall volume of 75 µl is reached each time. All material and products were stored on ice the entire time.

5. For the SOD standard curve, SOD standard was thawed on ice. Seven 1.5 ml micro tubes were numbered from one to seven. Then 620 µl 1x SOD buffer were added to tube 1, 100 µl 1x SOD buffer to tube 2,4,5 and 7, 150 µl 1x SOD buffer to tube 3 and 6. Afterwards, 5 µl SOD standard were added to tube 1 and vortexed well, then 100 µl were transferred from tube 1 to tube 2 and vortexed again, this step was repeated for the following tubes, always adding 100 µl from the previous tube to the next one plus vortexing in between. Thereby obtaining activities of 10 U/25 µl, 5 U/25 µl, 2 U/25 µl, 1 U/25 µl, 0.5 U/25 µl, 0.2 U/25 µl and 0.1 U/25 µl. Again all materials and products were stored on ice the entire time.

6. Once everything was prepared, 25 µl of 1x SOD buffer was added to every well.

Material and methods

7. 25 µl of each SOD standard dilution was added to the first 7 wells, leaving the last one empty. Then 25 µl of each sample solution were added to the remaining wells. This was done twice to obtain double results which were averaged.
8. Afterwards all wells have been filled up with 150 µl Master Mix using a multichannel pipet.
9. After booting the ELISA Reader plus software the 25 µl of 1x Xanthine solution was added to each well as a starter solution. After shaking the microtiter plate tenderly for 5 s, the plate was transferred immediately to the ELISA Reader and started the initial read with an absorbance of 450 nm every minute for 10 minutes at room temperature.

Procedure data interpretation:

1. To determine rate of change in absorbance. Duplicated absorbance values at 450 nm of the SOD Standard dilution series were averaged and plotted on the Y axis versus time in minutes on the X axis. The slope of each curve, change in absorbance at 450 nm per minute, was taken, resulting in the change in absorbance at 450 nm as a function of time.
2. The percentage of inhibition of the rate of change in absorbance at 450 nm was determined. The slope obtained in the absence of SOD, the Activity Control, should be maximal and was taken as the 100% value. All other slopes generated with SOD standards or *C. elegans* samples were compared to it. The % inhibition of the rate of increase in absorbance at 450 nm was calculated as follows:

$$\% \ Inhibition = \frac{[(Slope \ of \ 1x \ SOD \ Buffer \ Control) - (Slope \ of \ Sample)] \times 100}{(Slope \ of \ 1x \ Buffer \ Control)}$$

3. Considering that the SOD standard was provided at a concentration of 400 ng/µl with an activity of about 50 units/µl, the % Inhibition versus Log [units/well SOD standard] was plotted.
4. Then the % Inhibition of every *C. elegans* sample was related to the % Inhibition on the plot obtained one step previously thus obtaining the Log [units/well SOD standard] for the % Inhibition of the sample. The SOD specific activity and SOD concentration in the sample extract were derived as follows:

$$SOD \ specific \ activity = \frac{Anti \log(Sample \ related \ \% \ Inhib. \ of \ \log[units \ / \ well \ SOD \ stand.]}{amount \ of \ protein \ of \ investigated \ sample \ in \ \mu g}$$

$$SOD \ conc. \ in \ extract = SOD \ specific \ activity \ (units \ / \ \mu l) \times Protein \ conc. \ of \ sample \ (\mu g \ / \ \mu l)$$

2.2.5 BCA assay

For determining protein concentration of worm lysates the following protocol was used [183].

Protocol – BCA Assay in *C. elegans*:

Equipment and reagents:

- Clear microtiter plates uncoated
- ddH$_2$O
- BSA Standard 1 mg/ml
- BCA Staining Solution (1 volume share 4% CuSO$_4$ + 49 volume shares BCA)
- Eppendorf tubes 1.5 ml
- Precision Pipets ranging 10 to 1000 µl
- ELISA Reader plus Software
- Microsoft Excel 2003
- *C. elegans* lysates

Procedure:

1. A BSA Standard dilution series was created twice by using 1 mg/ml BSA stocks stored in aliquots at -20 °C, obtaining dilutions of 1:200, 1:100, 1:67, 1:40, 1:20, 1:13 and 1:10.
2. *C. elegans* homogenates were diluted 1:50, 1:100, 1:200, 1:400 and 1:800 with ddH$_2$O and protein concentration was determined in duplicates.
3. Using a microtiter plate, 100 µl of each standard dilution or 100 µl of each sample dilution were pipeted per well.
4. 100 µl of BCA staining solution per each well used was added and the microtiter plate was incubated for 30 min at 80 °C in the dark and evaluated afterwards using an ELISA Reader (Elx 800, Bio-TEK Instruments).
5. Afterwards, the obtained values were used and interpreted as follows using Microsoft Excel 2003:
    a. For every duplicate of the BSA Standard and *C. elegans* sample dilution the mean concentration was calculated.
    b. Averaged values were used to calculate a linear growth function y = mx + b by "=INDEX(RGP(y_values;x_values);array)" using the amount of added BSA Standard to each well as y-values and the averaged values obtained above were used as x-values, leaving "constant" and "stats" option blank as well as "column" and "row" option, implying that the values were following a linear growth pattern. For calculating the "m" value using "1" for describing the partial "array" of the y-values and using "2" for calculating the "b" value for describing the partial "array" of the x-values.
    c. Using the obtained "m" and "b" values the averaged sample dilution value was entered for "x" multiplicated by the reciprocal value of the sample dilution and divided by 1000, thereby calculating "y", which was the protein concentration in

mg/ml. The average of the five obtained protein concentration values, one for each dilution, was then used as the final protein concentration of the *C. elegans* lysate.

2.2.6 Western blot

To approve the expression of PrP^C, western blot analysis was chosen, using published protocols as a guideline [37, 189]. Therefore *C. elegans* were prepared as described in chapter 2.2.1.7 under step (1.) to (7.) except for using ddH$_2$O instead of S Buffer. To denaturise the nematodes the supernatant was aspirated and discarded while adding SDS-PAGE buffer (incl. 4% SDS and 5% mercpatoehtanol) to apply a negative charge to each protein in proportion to its mass and to reduce disulfide bridges to free thiols. The mixture was then shaken by 1400 rpm at 99 °C and stored at -20 °C, after measuring the protein concentration using the BCA assay, to assure comparable protein amounts would be highlighted by western blot analysis. For identification of PrP^C in worm preparations, gel electrophoresis was supplemented by Magic Marker, recombinant prion protein (recPrP) and human PrP^C, conserved from human lymphocytes. While cleanliness of the trial was assured by running Roti Load, *C. elegans* preparations were separated by sodium duodecyl sulfate-polyacrylamide gel electrophoresis (SDS-PAGE) [112] at 0.5 mA/cm^2 for around 90 min and blotted to semidry polyvinylidene difluoride membranes at 0.9 mA/cm^2 for 45 min. For western blot detection, the membranes were blocked for 60 min in PBS (phosphate buffered saline, pH 7.4)-0.075% Tween 20, containing 5% dry milk and incubated with the specific primary antibody 6H4 overnight at 4 °C. These were washed twice the next day in PBS-0.075% Tween 20 for 3 min, and once in PBS only for again 3 min. followed by the respective secondary antibody, Polyclonal Goat Anti-Mouse. Immunoreactive proteins were visualized by enhanced chemiluminescence (ECL Plus system; Amersham Biosciences).

2.2.7 Fluorescent Visualization

2.2.7.1 Dye Fill

Dye filling is a technique to stain amphid and phasmid neurons, which are accumulated in the head and tail of the nematode [8]. In this context the staining is used to compare the neurological uptake of the dye in all *C. elegans* strains.

For staining with DiI fluorescence stock solutions of 2 mg/ml in dimethyl formamide were used, stored at -20 °C in a foil wrapped tube. Before use the stock was diluted 1:200 in M9 (3 g KH$_2$PO$_4$, 6 g Na$_2$HPO$_4$, 5 g NaCl, 1 ml of 1 M MgSO$_4$, dissolved in 1 L of ddH$_2$O, stored at 4 °C). After transfusing 150 µl diluted stain to a microtiter well, around 20 worms were transferred into the dye and incubated at RT for 2 h. Worms were then transferred to a fresh NGM plate to let them crawl on a fresh bacterial lawn for about 1 h to destain the coverings and intestinal tract. For microscopic visualization worms were then transferred on 4% agarose pads, fixed with sodium azide and a coverslip which was sealed with conventional nail varnish. Visualization was obtained by using the Axio scope microscope (Zeiss) with Texas red filter (absorption wavelength: 596 nm; emission wavelength: 620 nm).

2.2.7.2 GFP visualisation

The green fluorescent protein (GFP) was translated from the transformed plasmids either with or without PrP^C sequence, therefore being a selective marker for successful transformation.

For this procedure worms were picked from NGM plates, transferred to 4% agarose pads and prepared as in 2.2.7.1. To conserve colorization a drop of SlowFade® was added to each gel pad. They were visualized by using the Axio scope microscope (Zeiss) with DAPI filter (absorption wavelength: 358 nm; emission wavelength: 461 nm).

A different preparation by shock freezing worms being investigated by liquid N_2 was considered to be obsolete, since GFP was possible to be visualized without destroying the nematodes cuticula.

2.2.8 Statistics

All statistics and graphs were done by Systat Software SigmaPlot 10.0 provided by ask|net AG or in rare cases by Microsoft Office Excel 2003.

For all lifespan tests, with or without stressors, log rank analysis was used to statistically evaluate the Kaplan-Meier curves with the Holm-Sidak method used to analyze multiple curves. Significant differences were proven by p-values, and critical level while significance level was not directly considered as the classical significance barrier (< 0.05). Critical level was calculated out of significance level and test distribution. If the p-value was smaller than critical level the null hypothesis was rejected, while a smaller critical level than significance level underlines the degree of significance [63].

3 Results

3.1 GFP fluorescence

The green fluorescent protein (GFP) is expressed either for selection purpose upon transformation with *hmg-12::gfp* or to indicate PrP^C expression after transformation with *Psel-12::huPrPc*.

In Figure 4 all lines which we have been working with were tested for the green fluorescent protein. All lines carrying a plasmid also ubiquitarily express the protein and gleam under DAPI filter, while those not expressing GFP, as there are wildtype, SOD-1 knock-out line and DAF-16 knock-out line, do not. All lines, however, also show a discreet natural auto-fluorescence, as seen in particular in wildtype after being illuminated for 600 ms and must not be confused with the artificial fluorescence caused by GFP. The different worms also show a different brightness or intensity of fluorescence, and this can be explained best by the different stages in growth or development, and by the number of embryos they are carrying; hence those do not gleam yet.

In Figure 5 the GFP gene was directly linked to the *Prnp* gene by inserting it into the protein itself in the SmaI-site of the gene so that functional and signal sequences were not harmed, to visualize the location of PrP^C expression. (A) and (B) show the head region of an adult worm each in which the problem is faced that the auto-fluorescence of the digestive tract almost outshines the GFP pattern, but it also clearly illustrates a fluorescence in many intracellular vesicles which are used to transport protein to and from membranes. Some GFP fluorescence is also seen in the membranes, but visualization was technically hardly to achieve because of minimal fluorescence and a short time frame to visualize and photograph the spot. In picture (C) an embryo is seen with dark cell nuclei and white frames, which mostly accord with the endoplasmatic reticulum. Those pictures were supplied by PD Dr. rer. nat. Schulze with whom existed a very close cooperation.

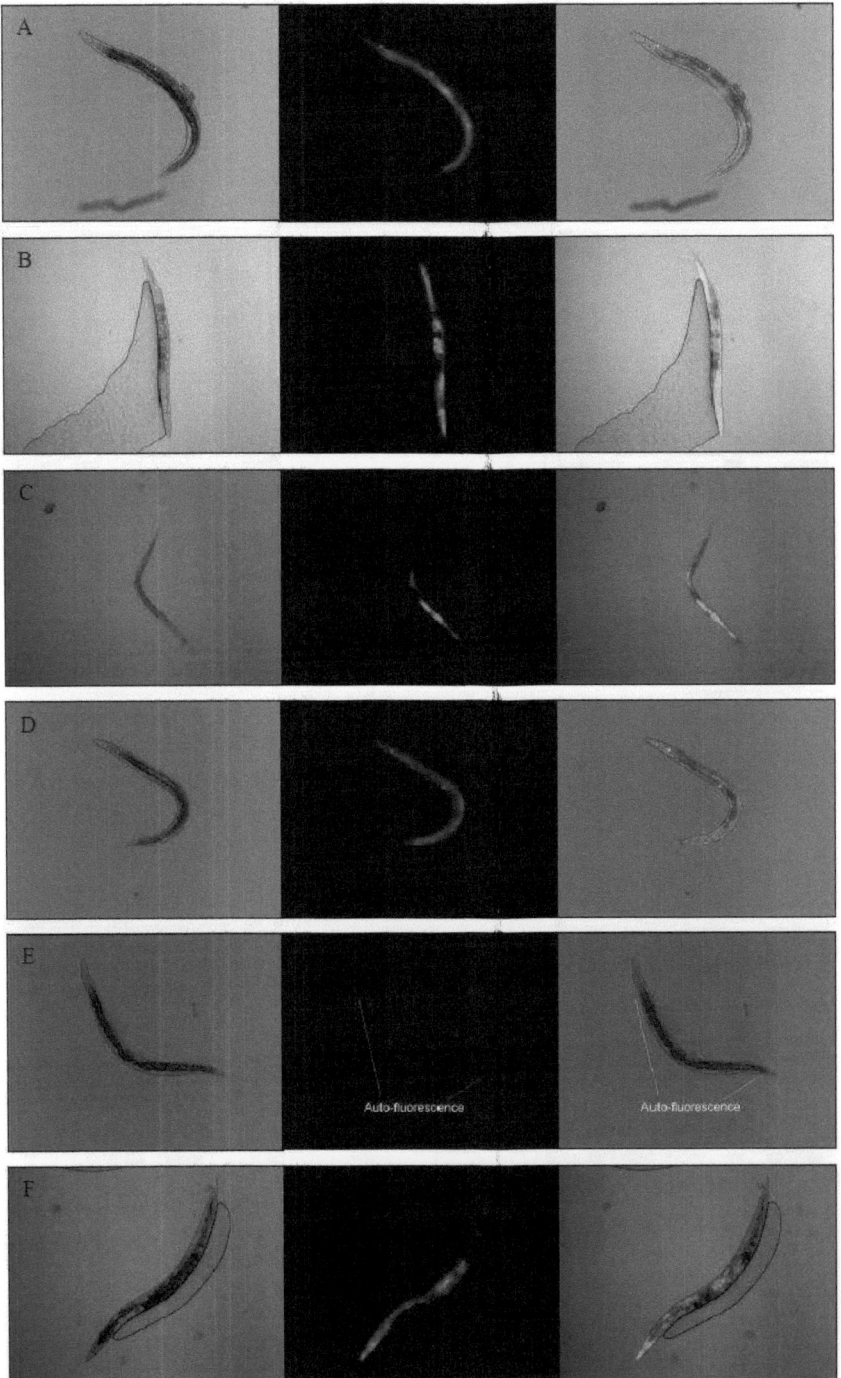

Results

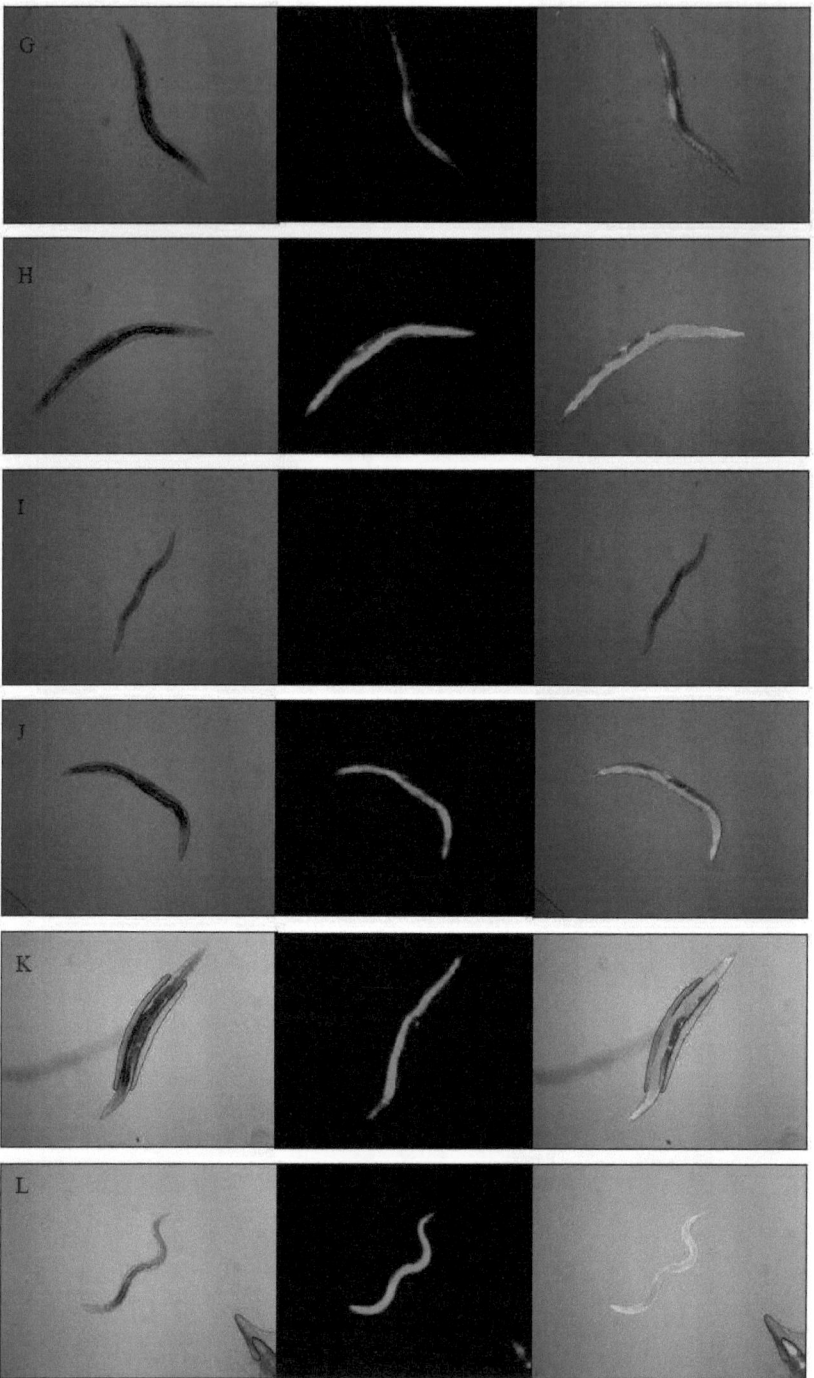

45

Figure 4: GFP Fluorescence
Left images are visualized with a standard filter, middle ones with a DAPI filter, right ones show left and middle images digitally stacked on top of each other. Illumination time was at 600 ms magnification 100x. (A) PrP line 1; (B) PrP line 2; (C) Octapeptide deleted Δ8; (D) plasmid line; (E) Wildtype with auto-fluorescence; (F) DAF-16 knock-out PrP line 2; (G) DAF-16 knock-out PrP line 1; (H) DAF-16 knock-out plasmid line; (I) DAF-16 knock-out line; (J) SOD-1 knock-out PrP line 2; (K) SOD-1 knock-out PrP line 1; (M) SOD-1 knock-out line; (L) SOD-1 knock-out plasmid line.

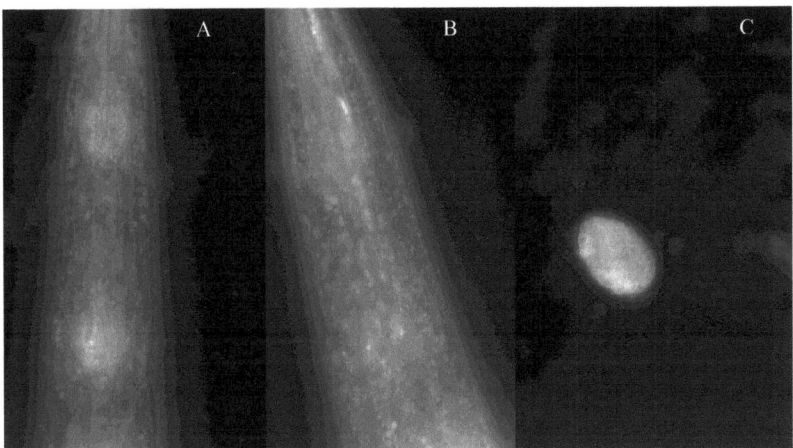

Figure 5: GFP-PrP^C linkage
GFP gene has been linked to *Prnp* to illustrate the location of PrP^C expression. (A) and (B) showing the head of an adult each, (C) showing an embryo. (A) and (B) mostly showing an PrP^C expression in intracellular vesicles, (C) in the endoplasmatic reticulum surrounding the dark cell nuclei. Pictures supplied by PD Dr. rer. nat. Schulze, working in close cooperation (Zeiss Axiomager Z1, Plan Apochromat 63x/1.40 Oil, Zeiss GFP Filter).

3.2 Western blot

Additionally, to the control for successful transformation, PCR was applied by our colleagues in Freiburg, who generated all used lines analyzed herein. Western blotting was done to control expression of PrP^C in those strains which were supposed to do so, as well as the absence in counter strains which should have been free of prion protein PrP^C. Only strains in long use were tested, since only those were in danger of genetical aberrations or genetical contaminations, hence SOD-4 and SOD-5 strains were not tested since their use was limited to less than five generations each after initial acquisition.

Figure 6 illustrates all long term *C. elegans* strains which were used, with a Magic Mark used as a kilo Dalton grid, lymphocytes achieved from human blood products as a huPrP^C source and recPrP to show the unglycolysated PrP^C. It can be seen that all lines which are supposed to express PrP^C also show bands in the frame of 20 to 40 kDa if labelled by PrP^C specific 6HA antibody, and those which should not do so also do not show any. Moreover, all Strains expressing prion protein show several bands representing prion protein products of different sizes.

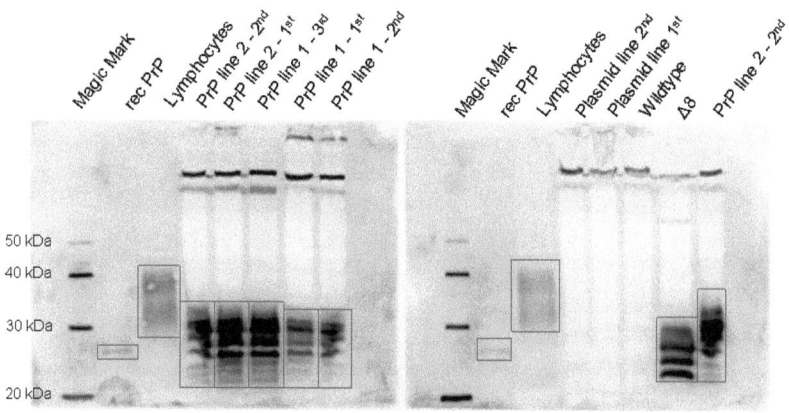

Results

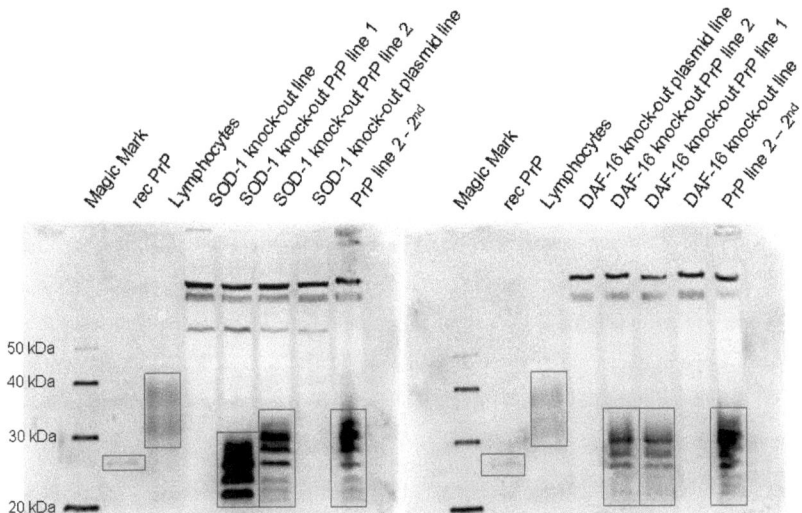

Figure 6:   PrP^C Western blot to control for PrP^C expression

Representative Western blots show three versions of PrP line 1 and two versions of PrP line 2 and plasmid line, which are genetically identical, but were chronologically picked at different times during a one year time frame, with 1st being the oldest and 3rd for PrP line 1 and 2nd for PrP line 2 and plasmid line being the most recent. Magic Mark is used as a kilo Dalton grid, showing bands at 20, 30, 40 and 50 kDa. Human lymphocytes serve as a comparison for huPrP^C it shows smooth blurry bands between 30 and 40 kDa and rec PrP shows a band at around 28 kDa, both in all for graphs. PrP line 2 1st and 2nd, PrP line 1 1st till 3rd, SOD-1 knock-out PrP line 1, SOD-1 knock-out PrP line 2, DAF-16 knock-out PrP line 2, and DAF-16 knock-out PrP line 1 all show an almost identical pattern of bands between ca. 35 kDa and 22 kDa for various prion protein products. While 1st and 2nd plasmid line, wildtype, SOD-1 knock-out line, SOD-1 knock-out plasmid line, DAF-16 knock-out plasmid line and DAF-16 knock-out line show no bands.

6H4 antibody 1:5000 first for overnight incubation at 4 °C, Goat-Anti-Mouse antibody 1:4000 second for 1 h at RT. All prion protein related bands are framed in a red box.

3.3 Lifespan determination

3.3.1 Prion protein expression vs. non-expression

Since the main objective of the experiment was to illuminate the physiologic function of PrP^C, several different genotypes were generated as listed in 2.1.1. The principle behind this is to have two different worm lines, one expressing PrP^C and one not. As *C. elegans* naturally does not express PrP^C this was artificially done by inserting a plasmid with *PRNP* being connected to the ubiquitously expressed promoter *sel-12*. In reality, this implicates four major lines, wildtype (N2), plasmid line (EC418) and PrP lines 1 (EC410) and 2 (EC411) both carrying prion protein encoding sequences, containing plasmid and expressing PrP^C.

One standard approach to investigate the phenotype of different genotypes is to carry out a lifespan determination. In this test the survival characteristics under non-hazardous standard laboratory conditions were obtained. Worms were kept at 25 °C at all times to ensure *pha-1* selection, dishes were checked for dead worms every 24 h and counted by testing for pharyngeal pumping.

Figure 7 identifies that controls, namely wildtype and plasmid line as well as PrP line 1 and 2 show a very similar lifespan pattern. Wildtype and plasmid line show, at a stage of 50% survival, a higher fitness (median lifespan: + 2 d) compared to PrP line 1 and 2.

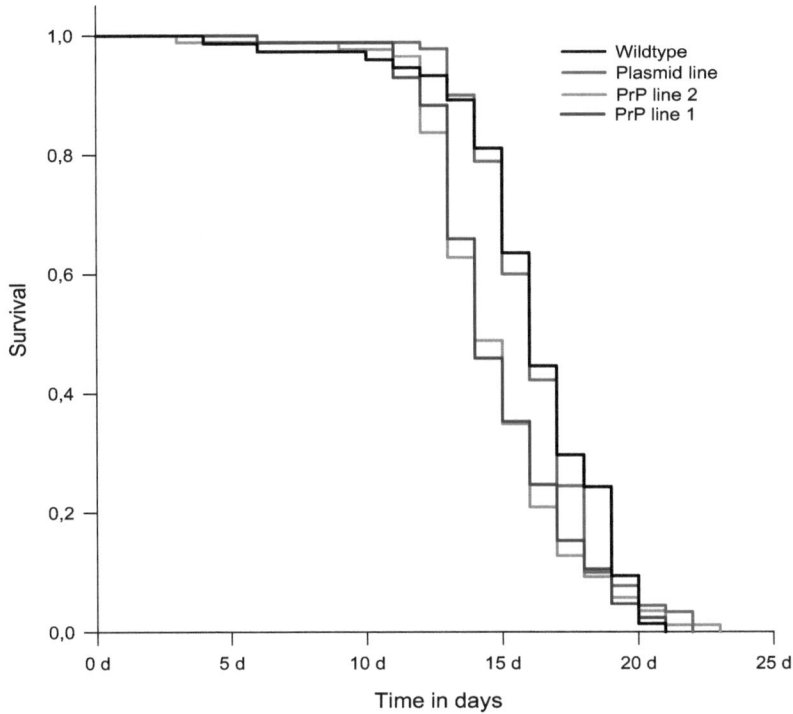

Figure 7:
Lifespan of PrP^C expressing vs. non-expressing strains
Plot showing the survival characteristics of wildtype (n = 74), plasmid line (n = 90) and PrP line 2 (n = 86) and PrP line 1 (n = 85). Wildtype compared to plasmid line identifies no statistically significant difference (p = 0.570; critical level = 0.00851). PrP line 1 compared to PrP line 2 identifies no statistically significant difference (p = 0.922; critical level = 0.0500). Wildtype compared to PrP line 1 (p = 0.00146; critical level = 0.00341) and to PrP line 2 (p = 0.00138; critical level = 0.00320) showing a statistically significant difference. Plasmid control line compared to PrP line 1 (p = 0.00200; critical level = 0.00394) and to PrP line 2 (p = 0.00244; critical level = 0.00427) showing a statistical significant difference. Mean lifespan being 14.7 d (Std. = 0.3) for PrP line 2, 16.1 d (Std. = 0.3) for plasmid line, 14.8 d (Std. = 0.3) for PrP line 1 and 16.1 d (Std. = 0.3) for wildtype.
Significance level = 0.05. Y-axis showing the relative population size from 0.0 to 1.0; x-axis showing the time frame in days.

Hence in Figure 7 it looks like the difference between wildtype, plasmid line and PrP line 1 and 2 is not based on a slower decrease in the population size, but actually on an earlier start in dying, which becomes neutralized by PrP line 1 and PrP line 2 by slowing the dying phase down after crossing the 50% mark of the population size, and the raw data was fitted in a sigmoidal plot to improve visualization, as it is seen in Figure 8. To further investigate the rate or speed of dying, the derivative of these sigmoidal curves in Figure 8 was created in Figure 9 where it becomes obvious that the statistical significant difference is not achieved by a difference in the speed of dying but rather in the onset of the dying phase.

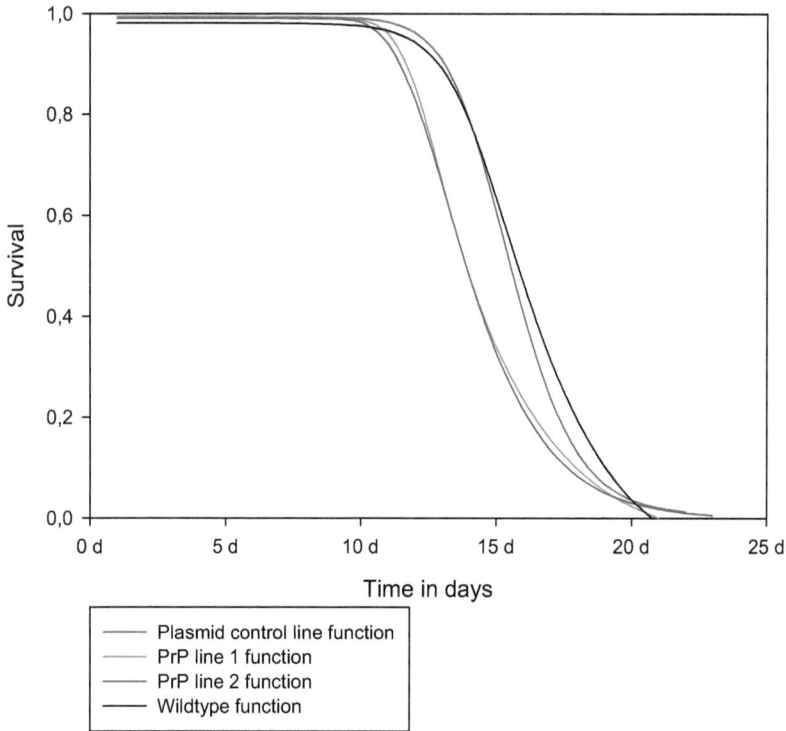

Figure 8: Sigmoidal fitting of lifespan data
Data from Figure 4 is fitted into a sigmoidal equation $y = a/(1+e^{-((X-X_0)/b)})$ to visually enhance the connection of wildtype and plasmid line, as well as PrP line 1 and PrP line 2 and to highlight the reason for the statistically significant difference in lifespan being caused by the onset of dying instead of the rate of dying.
Y-axis showing the relative population size from 0.0 to 1.0; x-axis showing the time frame in days.

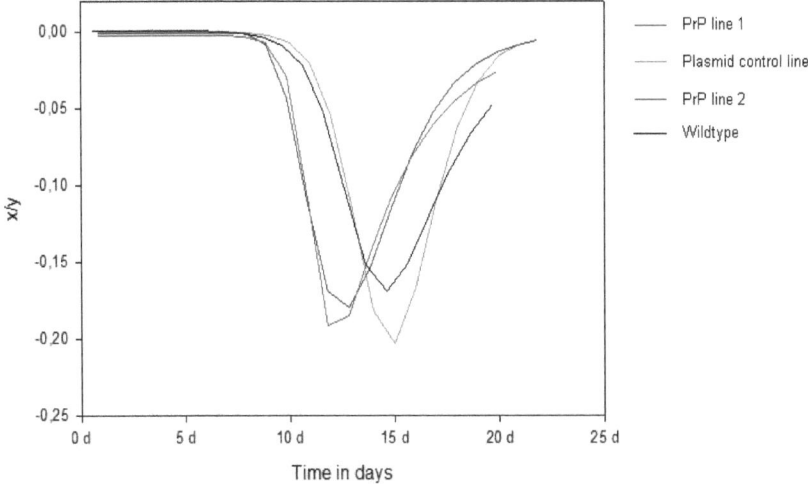

Figure 9: Speed of dying
Figure showing the first derivative of the sigmoid functions of Figure 8, therefore illustrating the speed of population decline, i.e. the speed of dying. PrP line 1 and PrP line 2 start off at around day 8 while wildtype and plasmid line start off at around day 10. All four lines have their maximum decline rate between -0.14 and -0.16.
Y-axis showing the speed of population decline per day starting with a whole of one; x-axis showing time in days starting at day zero.

3.3.2 DAF-16 / FoxO knock-out

To investigate a possible interaction of PrP^C with *C. elegans'* anti-stress responses, a DAF-16/FoxO deleted line was transformed with prion protein and tested. DAF-16, with its human homolog FoxO, being a nuclear transcription factor and the final effector of *daf-2* (an insulin/insulin like growth factor/receptor homolog) cellular stress response pathway, it was investigated if the absence of DAF-16/FoxO by knock-out shows an influence on lifespan characteristics compared to those expressing DAF-16/FoxO in figure 7 (3.3.1). Figure 10 compares DAF-16/FoxO knock-out lines with the lifespan behavior of wildtype out of figure 7. There is no statistically significant difference between DAF-16 knock-out PrP line 1 and DAF-16 knock-out PrP line 2, DAF-16 knock-out plasmid line, and DAF-16 knock-out line, but a significant decrease in lifespan of those compared to wildtype. Also, as in 3.3.1, an observed effect of an earlier onset in dying in prion protein expressing strains is no longer recognizable in DAF-16/FoxO knock-out strains.

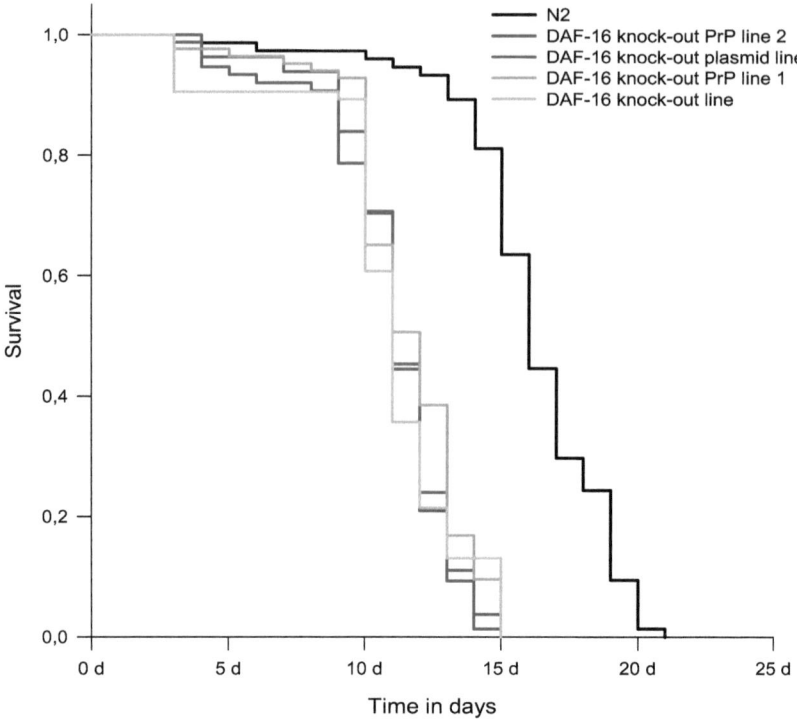

Figure 10: Lifespan FoxO/DAF-16 knock-out

Diagram showing wildtype (n = 74), DAF-16 knock-out PrP line 2 (n = 81) and DAF-16 knock-out PrP line 1 (n = 83), DAF-16 knock-out plasmid line (n = 75) and DAF-16 knock-out line (n = 84). There are no statistically significant differences between DAF-16 knock-out plasmid line and DAF-16 knock-out PrP line 2 (p = 0.834; critical level = 0.0253), DAF-16 knock-out PrP line 1 (p = 0.0525; critical level = 0.00394), DAF-16 knock-out line (p = 0.597; critical level = 0.00639). No statistically significant differences between DAF-16 knock-out PrP line 2 and DAF-16 knock-out PrP line 1 (p = 0.0895; critical level = 0.00427), DAF-16 knock-out line (p = 0.792; critical level = 0.0127). No statistically significant differences between DAF-16 knock-out PrP line 1 and DAF-16 knock-out line (p = 0.275; critical level = 0.00465). There are statistically significant differences between wildtype and DAF-16 knock-out plasmid line (p = 2.099E-28, critical level = 0.00101), DAF-16 knock-out PrP line 2 (p = 3.073E-28, critical level = 0.00103), DAF-16 knock-out PrP line 1 (p = 1.62E-25; critical level = 0.00114). Mean lifespan being 10.7 d (Std. = 0.2) for DAF-16 knock-out PrP line 2, 10.9 d (Std. = 0.3) for DAF-16 knock-out plasmid line, 11.5 d (Std. = 0.3) for DAF-16 knock-out PrP line 1, 10.8 d (Std. = 0.3) for DAF-16 knock-out line and 16.1 d (Std. = 0.3) for wildtype.

Significance level = 0.05. Y-axis showing the relative population size from 0.0 to 1.0; x-axis showing the time frame in days.

3.3.3 SKN-1/Nrf-2 modification by RNAi

With SKN-1 being a transcription factor for phase II reaction enzymes, and Nrf-2 being its human homolog, it is the final target of p38-MAPK cellular stress pathway and object of investigation as a possible interactor for PrP^C. Therefore SKN-1/Nrf-2 ribosomal translation was inhibited in prion protein expressing and non-expressing lines by complementary RNAi as described in 2.2.1.3, and its lifespan characteristics were compared with wildtype as it is seen in figure 11.

The results of SKN-1/Nrf-2 inhibition are very similar to those of DAF-16/FoxO knock-out in figure 10. Compared to the median lifespan of all DAF-16/FoxO knock out lines (11 days), in SKN-1/Nrf-2 inhibition lines it is elongated by one day (12 days) but still four days shorter than wildtype (16 days). Similar to DAF-16/FoxO knock-out, the observed effect seen in 3.3.1 of an earlier onset in dying of the prion protein expressing strains was no longer possible to monitor.

Results

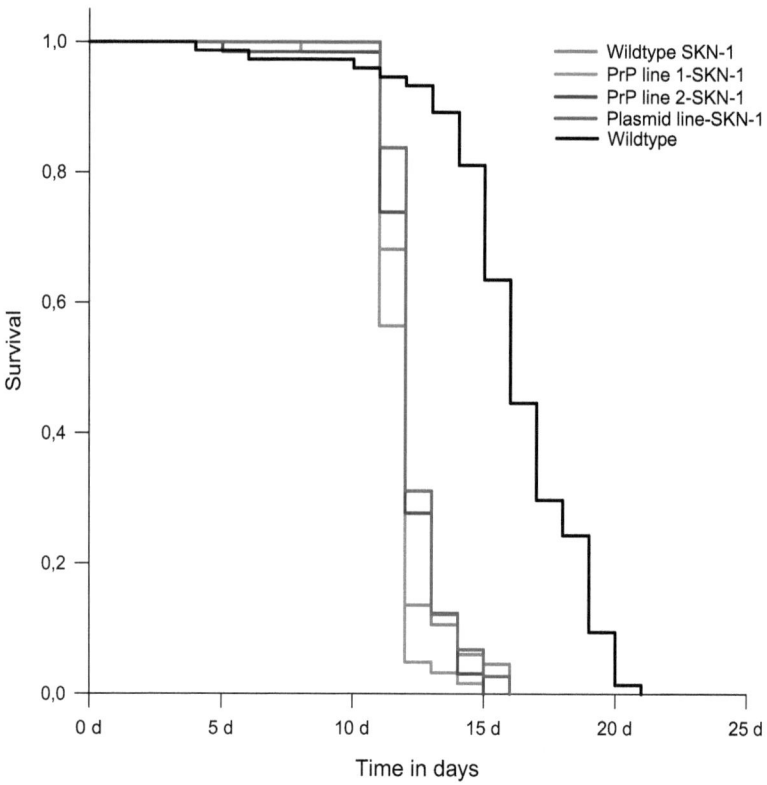

Figure 11: Lifespan of SKN-1/Nrf-2 inhibition by RNAi

Diagram showing plasmid line-SKN-1 (n = 74), PrP line 2-SKN-1 (n = 65) and PrP line 1-SKN-1 (n = 62), wildtype-SKN-1 (n = 66) modified by RNAi to inhibit SKN-1 translation plus wildtype (n = 74) as comparison. Plasmid line-SKN-1 showing no statistically significant difference to PrP line 2-SKN-1 (p = 0.236; critical level = 0.00851), wildtype-SKN-1 (p = 0.0921; critical level = 0.00568). No statistically significant difference between PrP line 1-SKN-1 and wildtype-SKN-1 (p = 0.681; critical level = 0.0253). There is statistically significant difference between PrP line 1-SKN-1 and plasmid line-SKN-1(p = 0.0000162; critical level = 0.00341), PrP line 2-SKN-1 (p = 0.00317; critical level = 0.00394) but no statistically significant difference between PrP line 1-SKN-1 and wildtype-SKN-1 (p = 0.0339; critical level = 0.00465). Statistically significant difference between wildtype and plasmid line-SKN-1 (p = 7.779E-24; critical level = 0.00285), PrP line 2-SKN-1 (p = 4.22E-25; critical level = 0.00256), PrP line 1-SKN-1 (p = 1.744E-25; critical level = 0.00244), wildtype-SKN-1 (p = 2.984E-22; critical level = 0.00320). Mean lifespan being 12.0 d (Std. = 0.2) for wildtype-SKN-1, 11.6 d (Std. = 0.1) for PrP line 1-SKN-1, 12.1 d (Std. = 0.2) for PrP line 2-SKN-1, 12.4 d (Std. = 0.1) for plasmid line-SKN-1 and 16.1 d (Std. = 0.3) for wildtype.

Significance level = 0.05. Y-axis showing the relative population size from 0.0 to 1.0; x-axis showing the time frame in days.

3.3.4 SOD-1 knock-out

As SOD-1 is known as one of the major correcting variables of stress pathways, a part of the end products of the stress response systems has now been deleted instead of antecedent variables. In this lifespan study, figure 12, wildtype has been compared to a *sod-1* knock-out line.
SOD-1 shows no influence on lifespan behavior since SOD-1 knock-out line has an almost identical lifespan pattern than wildtype.

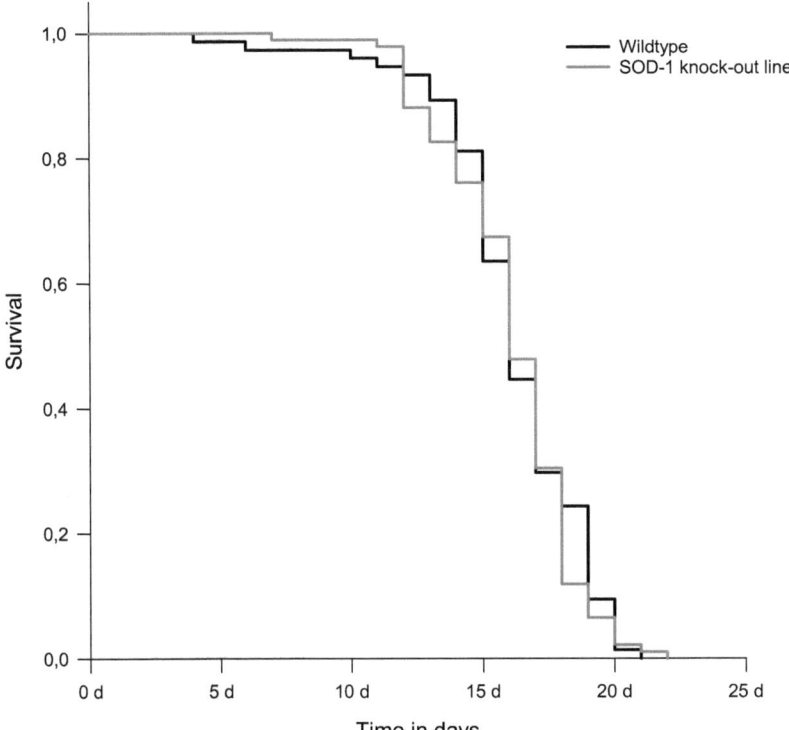

Figure 12: Lifespan SOD-1 knock-out
Diagram showing SOD-1 knock-out line (n = 92) and for comparison wildtype (n = 74). There is no statistically significant difference between SOD-1 knock-out line and wildtype (p = 0.631; critical level = 0.00851). Mean lifespan being 16.1 d (Std. = 0.4) for SOD-1 knock-out line and 16.1 d (Std. = 0.3) for wildtype.
Significance level = 0.05. Y-axis showing the relative population size from 0.0 to 1.0; x-axis showing the time frame in days.

3.3.5 Octarepeat deletion

The N-terminus of PrP^C is strongly associated with any function of the protein, especially residues 51-81, also known as the octarepeat region, hence it is a sequence of repeating octapeptides. Figure 13 illustrates the lifespan of a strain expressing a PrP^C which has its octarepeat region being deleted, the Δ8 worm. In comparison to wildtype it shows no statistically significant difference. The initial lifespan effect of PrP^C seen in figure 7 is not recognizable.

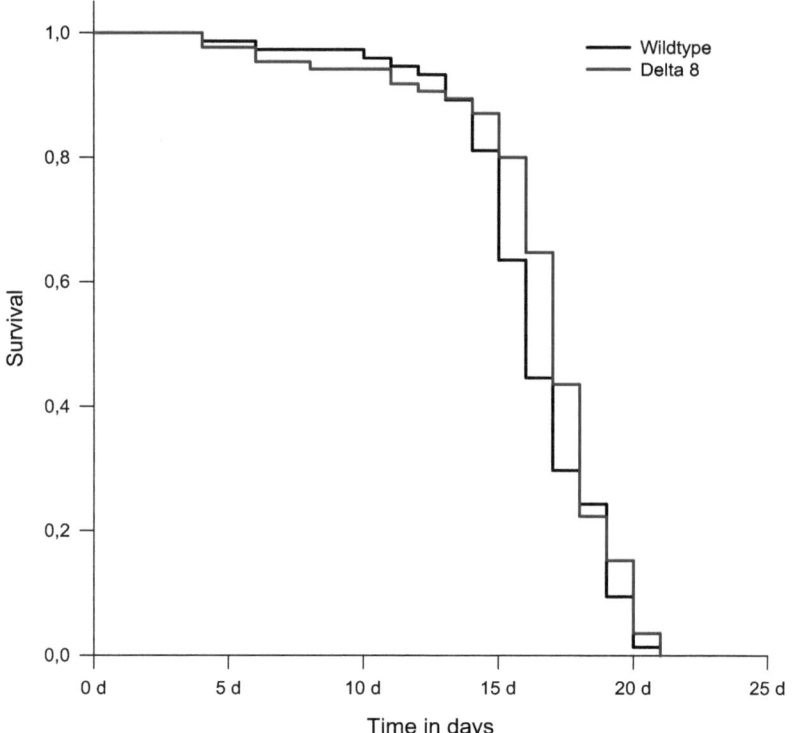

Figure 13: Lifespan Δ8
Diagram showing the lifespan characteristics of Δ8 (n = 85) in comparison to wildtype (n = 74). There is no statistically significant difference between them (p = 0.0855; critical level = 0.0500). Mean lifespan being 16.6 d (Std. = 0.4) for Δ8 and 16.1 d (Std. = 0.3) for wildtype.
Significance level = 0.05. Y-axis showing the relative population size from 0.0 to 1.0; x-axis showing the time frame in days.

3.4 Paraquat stress assays

3.4.1 Prion protein expression vs. non-expression

In this trial the resistance to superoxide anions produced by Paraquat, also known as Methylviologen, of PrP line 1 and PrP line 2 are compared to wildtype and plasmid line. Figure 14 illustrates the lifespan behavioral of the mentioned lines under oxidative stress caused by 100 mM Paraquat dissolved in NGM, showing that wildtype and plasmid line behave equally as well as PrP line 1 and PrP line 2. However, the curve also demonstrates a distinctive advantage in oxidative resistance of PrP line 1 and PrP line 2 compared to wildtype and plasmid line (e.g. mean lifespan being 6.7 h for wildtype and 10.5 h for PrP line 2).

Results

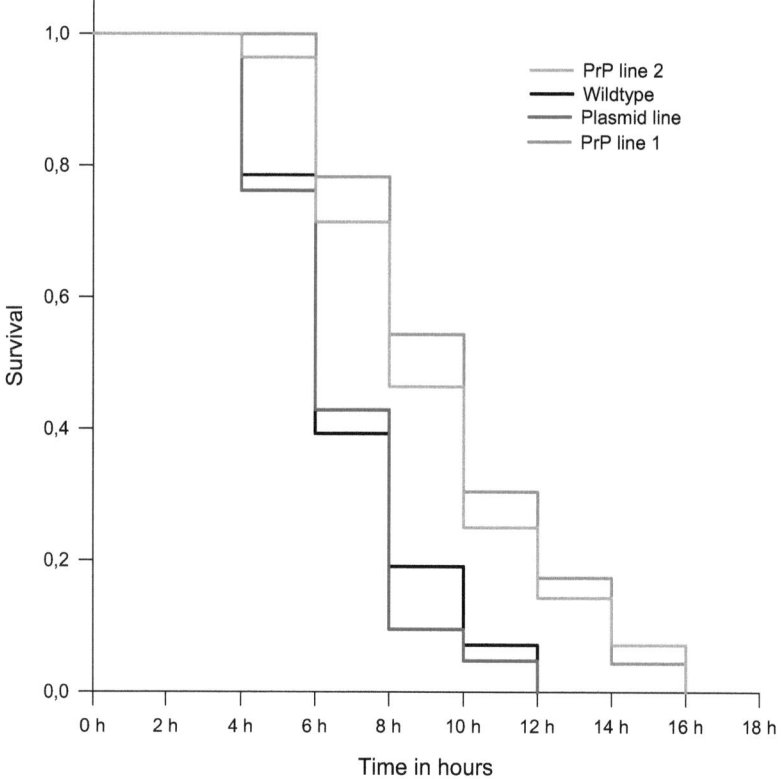

Time in hours

Figure 14: Lifespan under Paraquat of prion protein vs. no prion protein expressing strains
Diagram showing the lifespan characteristics of wildtype (n = 84), plasmid line (n = 42), PrP line 1 (n = 46) and PrP line 2 (n = 66) under permanent oxidative stress. There is no statistically significant difference between wildtype and plasmid line (p = 0.596; critical level = 0.0170), between PrP line 2 and PrP line 1 (p = 0.0791; critical level = 0.00394). There is a statistically significant difference between wildtype and PrP line 1 (p = 2.28E-7; critical level = 0.00155), PrP line 2 (p = 7.477E-11; critical level = 0.00135). There is statistically significant difference between plasmid line and PrP line 1 (p = 6.71E-7; critical level = 0.00171), EC 411 (p = 1.63E-9; critical level = 0.00142). Mean lifespan being 6.9 h (Std. = 0.3) for wildtype, 6.7 h (Std. = 0.3) for plasmid line, 10.5 h (Std. = 0.5) for PrP line 2, 9.7 h (Std. = 0.4) for PrP line 1.
Significance level = 0.05. Y-axis showing the relative population size; x-axis showing a time frame in hours.

Results

3.4.2 DAF-16/FoxO knock-out

With DAF-16/FoxO being the prominent part of major stress resistance pathways in *C. elegans*, PrP^C expressing lines with a deletion of DAF-16 were compared to DAF-16 deleted lines not expressing PrP^C while coping with Paraquat stress. Figure 15 illustrates a statistically significant difference in lifespan behavioral between DAF-16 knock-out PrP line 1, DAF-16 knock-out PrP line 2 and DAF-16 knock-out line, DAF-16 knock-out plasmid line, demonstrating an advantage for those expressing prion protein (e.g. mean lifespan being 8.1 h for DAF-16 knock-out plasmid line and 11.4 h for DAF-16 knock-out PrP line 1).

On the other hand, those lines not expressing PrP^C but with DAF-16/FoxO (wildtype, plasmid line) each show a significant disadvantage in Paraquat stress coping compared to their companions lacking DAF-16/FoxO expression (DAF-16 knock-out line, DAF-16 knock-out plasmid line), seen in figure 16. This phenomenon is not as clearly seen when those lines expressing Prion protein and DAF-16/FoxO (PrP line 1, PrP line 2) in figure 17 are compared to their companions missing DAF-16/FoxO expression (DAF-16 knock-out PrP line 1, DAF-16 knock-out PrP line 2) a statistically significant difference only being observed between PrP line 1 and DAF-16 knock-out PrP line 1, seen in figure 17. Although not significant, the difference in the other pair between PrP line 2 and DAF-16 knock-out PrP line 2 is still visible.

Figure 18 illustrates the difference in the rate of flight between *C. elegans* expressing DAF-16/FoxO and those being a knock-out for this nuclear factor. Flight is defined by those worms crawling up the edge of the petri dish to avoid Paraquat poisoning but thereby accepting death by exsiccation. Those lines lacking DAF-16/FoxO clearly had a lower intention of flight (16% - 24%) than those which were not (51% - 71%).

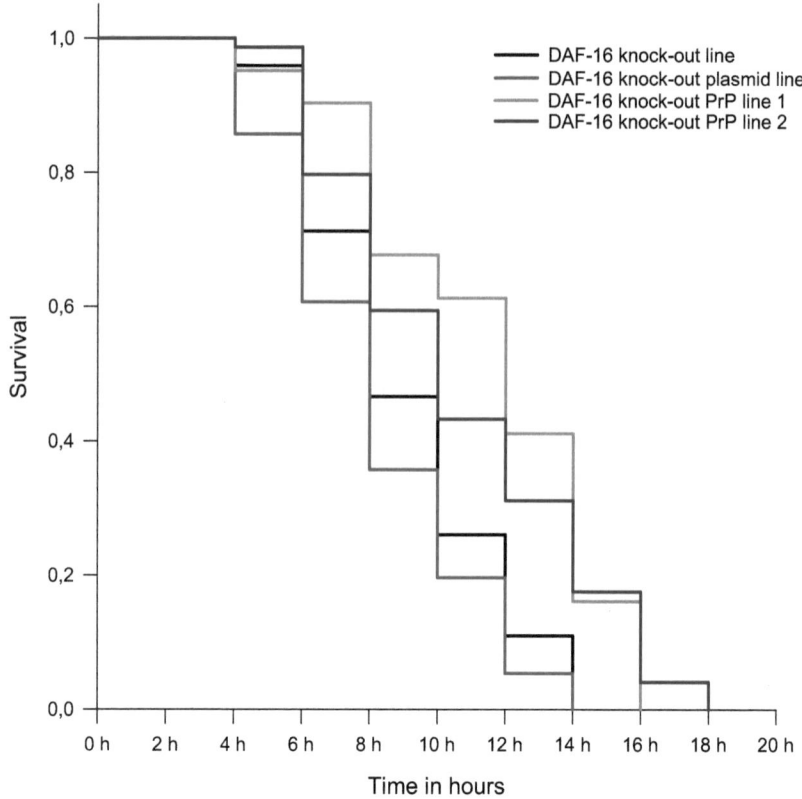

Figure 15: Lifespan under Paraquat of DAF-16/FoxO knock-out in PrP^C vs. no PrP^C expressing strains

Diagram showing DAF-16 knock-out PrP line 1 (n = 124) and DAF-16 knock-out PrP line 2 (n = 74), DAF-16 knock-out plasmid line (n = 112), and DAF-16 knock-out line (n = 146). No statistically significant difference between DAF-16 knock-out line and DAF-16 knock-out plasmid line (p = 0.0245; critical level = 0.00301), as well between DAF-16 knock-out PrP line 2 and DAF-16 knock-out PrP line 1 (p = 0.394; critical level = 0.0102). Statistically significant difference between DAF-16 knock-out line and DAF-16 knock-out PrP line 1 (p = 1.519E-011; critical level = 0.00128), DAF-16 knock-out PrP line 2 (p = 0.0000389; critical level = 0.00183), as well as between DAF-16 knock-out plasmid line and DAF-16 knock-out PrP line 2 (p = 0,000000308;critical level = 0.00160), DAF-16 knock-out PrP line 1 (p = 5.326E-015; critical level = 0.00119). Mean lifespan being 10.7 h (Std. = 0.4) for DAF-16 knock-out PrP line 2 and 11.4 h (Std. = 0.3) for DAF-16 knock-out PrP line 1, 9.0 h (Std. = 0.2) for DAF-16 knock-out line, 8.1 h (Std. = 0.3) for DAF-16 knock-out plasmid line.

Significance level = 0.05. Y-axis showing the relative population size; x-axis showing a time frame in hours.

Results

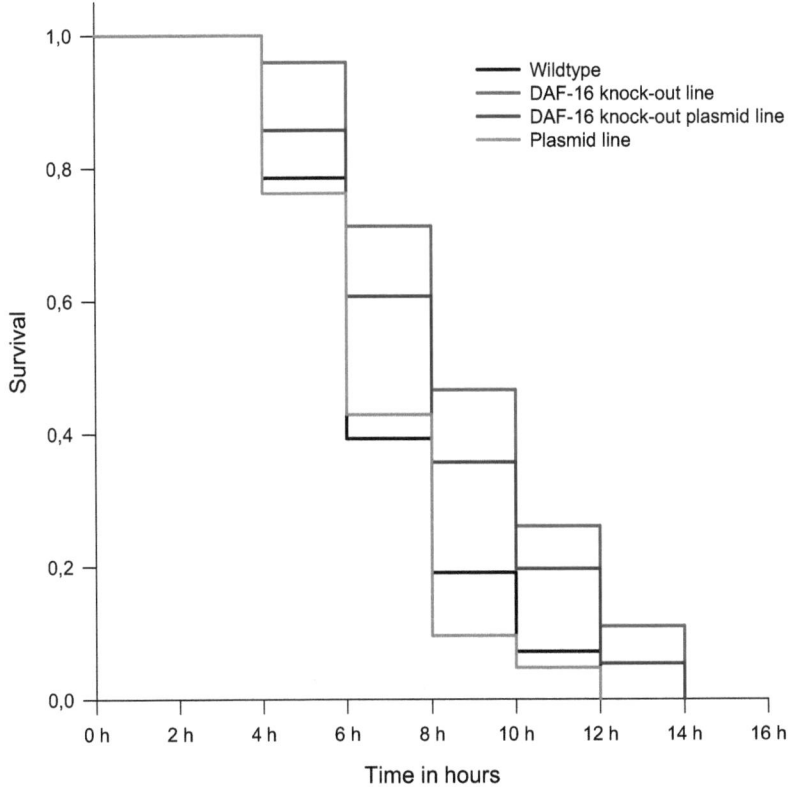

Figure 16: No prion protein with and without DAF-16/FoxO
Diagram showing wildtype (n = 84) and plasmid line (n = 42) plus its DAF-16/FoxO deleted companions DAF-16 knock-out line (n = 146) and DAF-16 knock-out plasmid line (n = 112). There is no statistically significant difference between wildtype and plasmid line (p = 0.596; critical level = 0.0170) as well between DAF-16 knock-out line and DAF-16 knock-out plasmid line (p = 0.0245; critical level = 0.00301). There is statistically significant difference between wildtype and DAF-16 knock-out line (p = 1.04E-8; critical level = 0.00146), DAF-16 knock-out plasmid line (p = 0.000667; critical level = 0.00233) as well between plasmid line and DAF-16 knock-out line (p = 2.18E-7; critical level = 0.00151), DAF-16 knock-out plasmid line (p = 0.00125; critical level = 0.00256). Mean lifespan being 6.9 h (Std. = 0.3) for wildtype, 9.0 h (Std. = 0.2) for DAF-16 knock-out line, 8.1 h (Std. = 0.3) for DAF-16 knock-out plasmid line and 6.7 h (Std. = 0.3) for plasmid line.
Significance level = 0.05. Y-axis showing the relative population size; x-axis showing a time frame in hours.

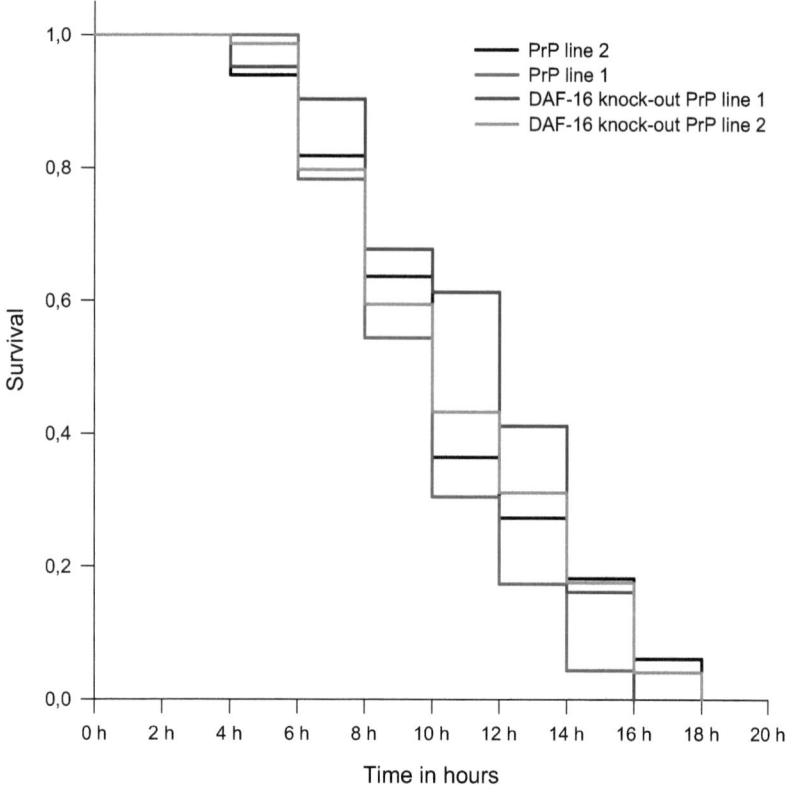

Figure 17: Prion protein expressing strains with and without DAF-16/FoxO
Diagram showing PrP line 2 (n = 66) and PrP line 1 (n = 46) plus its DAF-16/FoxO deleted companions DAF-16 knock-out PrP line 2 (n = 118) and DAF-16 knock-out PrP line 1 (n = 124). There is no statistically significant difference between PrP line 2 and PrP line 1 (p = 0.0791; critical level = 0.00394), DAF-16 knock-out PrP line 1 (p = 0.982; critical level = 0.0500), EC4905 (p = 0.371; critical level = 0.00851) as well between PrP line 1 and DAF-16 knock-out PrP line 2 (p = 0.0561; critical level = 0.00341). There is a statistically significant difference between PrP line 1 and DAF-16 knock-out PrP line 1 (p = 0.000479; critical level = 0.00223). Mean lifespan being 10.5 h (Std. = 0.5) for PrP line 2, 9.7 h (Std. = 0.4) for PrP line 1, 10.7 h (Std. = 0.4) for DAF-16 knock-out PrP line 2 and 11.4 h (Std. = 0.3) for DAF-16 knock-out PrP line 1. Significance level = 0.05. Y-axis showing the relative population size; x-axis showing a time frame in hours.

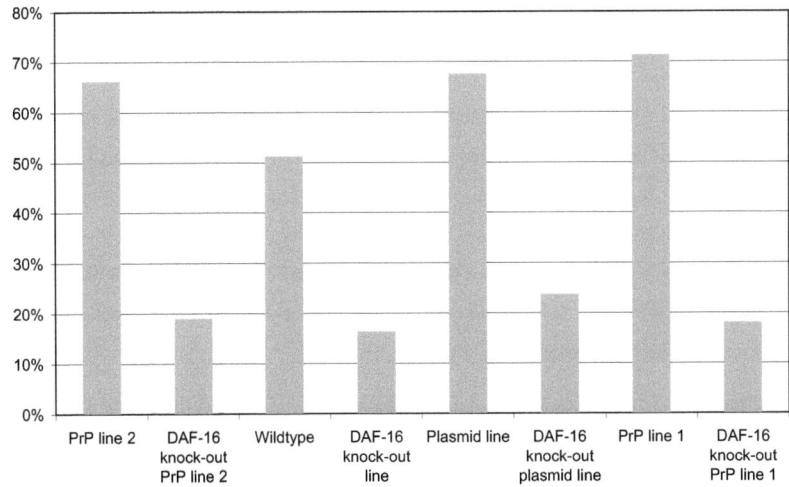

Figure 18: Flight rate during Paraquat exposure and DAF-16/FoxO knock-out

Diagram showing the different flight behavior of C. elegans with and without DAF-16/FoxO. It shows the number of worms in percent which try to leave the petri dish by climbing up the dish's wall which is inevitable connected with their death by exsiccation. PrP line 2 (n = 360) having a loss of 66%, DAF-16 knock-out PrP line 2 (n = 360) of 19%, wildtype (n = 262) of 51%, DAF-16 knock-out line (n = 160) of 16%, plasmid line (n = 160) of 68%, DAF-16 knock-out plasmid line (n = 220) of 24%, PrP line 1 (n = 160) of 71%, DAF-16 knock-out PrP line 1 (n = 240) of 18%.

Y-axis showing the relative rate of flight in percent; x-axis showing the different C. elegans lines.

3.4.3 SKN-1/Nrf-2 modification by RNAi

Similar to DAF-16/FoxO, SKN-1/Nrf-2 is a nuclear transcription factor and a prominent cornerstone of *C. elegans*' stress pathways. In this trial, prion protein expressing lines were compared with non-expressing while the SKN-1/Nrf-2 translation was inhibited on the tRNA level by complementary RNAi. Figure 19 illustrates that the inhibition of SKN-1/Nrf-2 does not change the relations previously illustrated with prion protein expressing lines (PrP line 2-SKN-1, PrP line 1-SKN-1) more resistant against Paraquat than those not expressing (wildtype-SKN-1, plasmid line-SKN-1) with statistically significant difference (e.g. mean lifespan being 14.7 h for PrP line 1-SKN-1 and 9.4 h for wildtype-SKN-1). Almost no resistance is seen in the line not expressing SOD-1 (SOD-1 knock-out line-SKN-1) (mean lifespan being 4.2 h).

Moreover, in figure 20, when wildtype and wildtype-SKN-1 as well as PrP line 1 and PrP line 1-SKN-1 are being compared, a several phenomena become obvious. Firstly, the SKN-1/Nrf-2 inhibition does not lead to a disadvantage, but actually to a benefit with a statistically significant difference. Secondly, the advantage of prion protein expressing during Paraquat exposure even further increases if SKN-1/Nrf-2 is inhibited, i.e. when the median lifespan is compared, the difference between no prion protein and prion protein increases from 4 hours to 6 hours when SKN-1/Nrf-2 is inhibited.

The loss from flight behavior, seen in figure 21, relatively converges between the different lines (51 – 71%) except for PrP line 1-SKN-1 (27%) and PrP line 2-SKN-1 (16%).

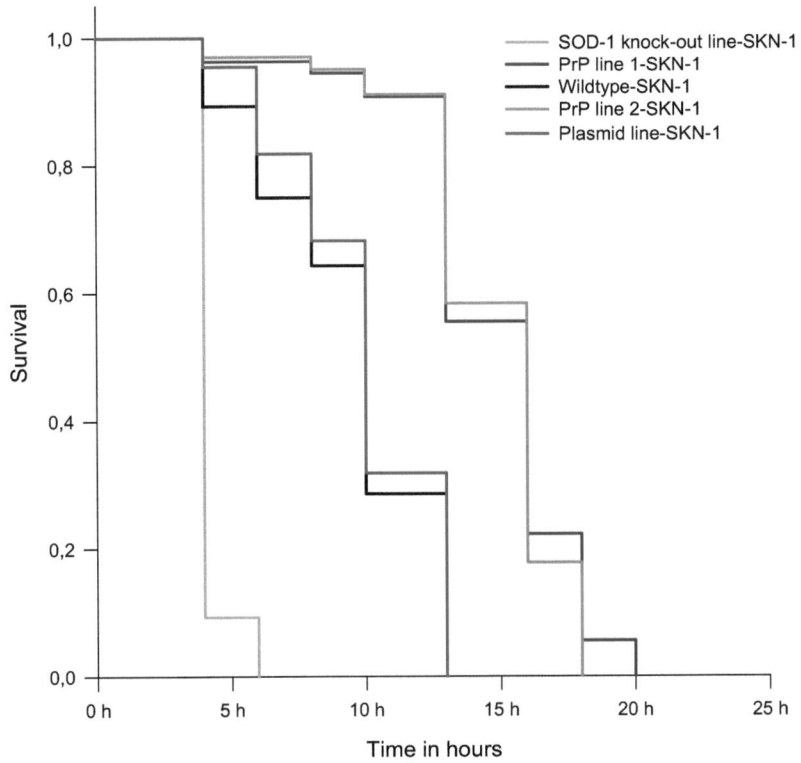

Figure 19: Lifespan under SKN-1 inhibition by RNAi in PrP^C vs. no PrP^C expressing strains
Diagram showing the different lifespan characteristics of *C. elegans* expressing prion protein and SOD-1 or not while inhibiting SKN-1. These are PrP line 1-SKN-1 (n = 108), PrP line 2-SKN-1 (n = 101), plasmid line-SKN-1 (n = 44), wildtype-SKN-1 (n = 56), SOD-1 knock-out line-SKN-1 (n = 108. There is no statistically significant difference between wildtype-SKN-1 and plasmid line-SKN-1 (p = 0.593; critical level = 0.0500), as well between PrP line 1-SKN-1 and PrP line 2-SKN-1 (p = 0.435; critical level = 0.0253). There is statistically significant difference between SOD-1 knock-out line-SKN-1 and PrP line 1-SKN-1 (p = 5.695E-50; critical level = 0.00341), PrP line 2-SKN-1 (p = 3.619E-49; critical level = 0.00366), plasmid line-SKN-1 (p = 4.498E-30; critical level = 0.00394), wildtype-SKN-1 (p = 9.485E-30; critical level = 0.00427), between PrP line 2-SKN-1 and plasmid line-SKN-1 (p = 1.506E-18; critical level = 0.00851), wildtype-SKN-1 (p = 1.325E-21; critical level = 0.00639), as well between PrP line 1-SKN-1 and wildtype-SKN-1 (p = 1.918E-21; critical level = 0.00730), plasmid line-SKN-1 (p = 2.898E-18; critical level = 0.0102. Mean lifespan being 14.7 h (Std. = 0.3) for PrP line 1-SKN-1, 9.4 h (Std. = 0.4) for wildtype-SKN-1, 14.6 h (Std. = 0.3) for PrP line 2-SKN-1, 9.9 h (Std. = 0.4) for plasmid line-SKN-1 and 4.2 h (Std. = 0.06) for SOD-1 knock-out line-SKN-1.
Significance level = 0.05. Y-axis showing the relative population size; x-axis showing a time frame in hours.

Results

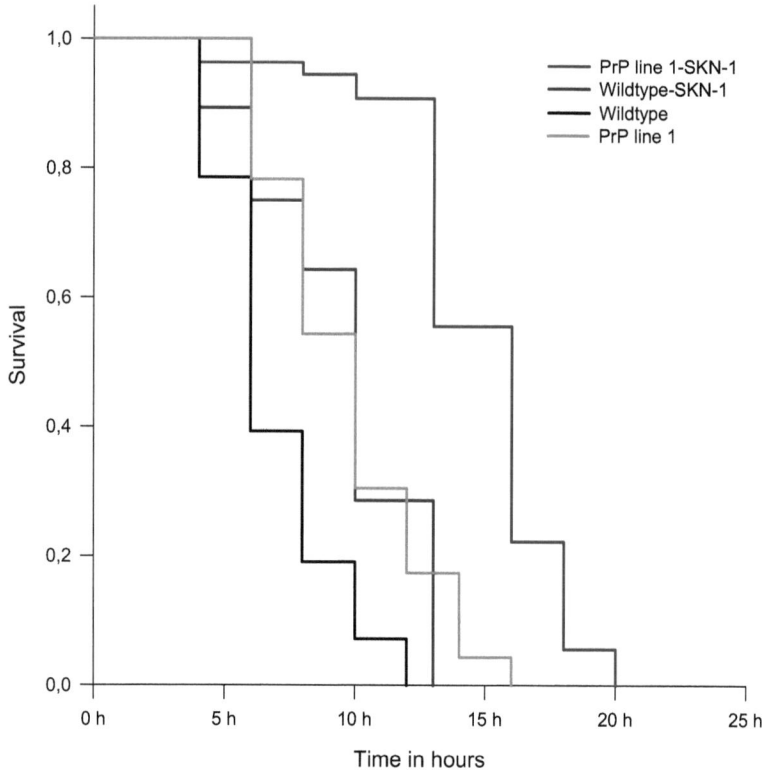

Figure 20: SKN-1 inhibition effect under Paraquat

Diagram showing wildtype plus PrP line 1 with and without SKN-1 inhibition, wildtype-SKN-1 (n = 56), PrP line 1-SKN-1 (n = 108), wildtype (n = 84), PrP line 1 (n = 46). There is a statistically significant difference between wildtype and wildtype-SKN-1 (p = 6.66E-9; critical level 0.00512), PrP line 1 (p = 2.28E-7; critical level = 0.00568), PrP line 1-SKN-1 (p = 9.548E-43, critical level = 0.00197) between PrP line 1 and PrP line 1-SKN-1 (p = 3.966E-20; critical level = 0.00341), between wildtype-SKN-1 and PrP line 1-SKN-1 (p = 1.918E-21; critical level = 0.00730). There is no statistically significant difference between PrP line 1 and wildtype-SKN-1 (p = 0.599; critical level = 0.0253). Mean lifespan being 14.7 h (Std. = 0.3) for PrP line 1-SKN-1, 9.4 h (Std. = 0.4) for wildtype-SKN-1, 6.9 h (Std. = 0.3) for wildtype and 9.7 h (Std. = 0.4) for PrP line 1.
Significance level = 0.05. Y-axis showing the relative population size; x-axis showing a time frame in hours.

Results

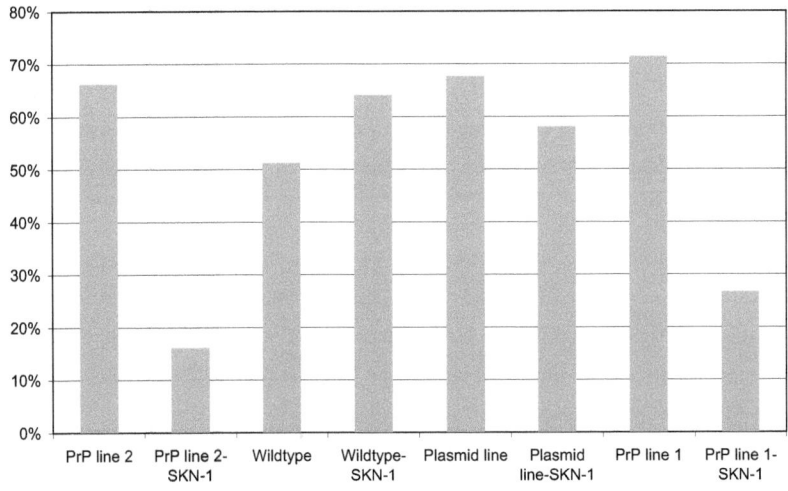

Figure 21: Flight rate during Paraquat exposure and SKN-1/Nrf-2 **inhibition**
Diagram showing the different flight behavior of C. elegans with and without SKN-1/Nrf-2 inhibition during Paraquat exposure. It shows the number of worms in percent which try to leave the petri dish by climbing up the dish's wall which is inevitable connected with their death by exsiccation. PrP line 2 (n = 360) having a loss of 66%, PrP line 2-SKN-1 (n = 75) of 16%, wildtype (n = 262) of 51%, wildtype-SKN-1 (n = 75) of 64%, plasmid line (n = 160) of 68%, plasmid line-SKN-1 (n = 50) of 58%, PrP line 1 (n = 160) of 71%, PrP line 1-SKN-1 (n = 75) of 27%.
Y-axis showing the relative rate of flight in percent; x-axis showing the different C. elegans lines.

3.4.4 SOD knock-out

Paraquat is a creator of superoxide anions $O_2^{\cdot -}$, and the superoxide dismutase (SOD), is responsible for deactivating this cellular hazard into H_2O_2, which then is decomposed further by subsequent enzymes. In this trial, prion protein expressing lines as well as non-expressing lines were modified by knocking out the different Cu^{2+}/Zn^{2+} SODs of *C. elegans* which are SOD-1, SOD-4 and SOD-5 and stressing them with Paraquat.

Figure 22 illustrates the effect of SOD-1 knock-out. All lines with a SOD-1 knock-out show an almost identical resistance pattern which leads to the death of almost any worm after four hours. There is no statistically significant difference between those knock-out lines. Compared to wildtype, those have a significantly shorter lifespan if stressed by Paraquat (mean lifespan being 3.2 – 3.5 hours in SOD-1 knock-out lines compared to 7.6 hours in wildtype).

The effect of SOD-5 knock-out is shown in figure 23. There is no statistically significant difference between wildtype and the SOD-5 knock-out lines, as well between prion protein expressing and non-expressing if stressed by Paraquat (Mean lifespan being 8.2 – 8.9 hours for all lines).

Figure 24 shows the effect of SOD-4 knock-out. On the one hand, SOD-4 knock-out lines have a similar Paraquat resistance pattern as plasmid line, showing no statistically significant difference. On the other hand, there is no statistical difference between SOD-4 knock-out lines expressing prion protein and those which do not (all mean lifespan being between 9.9 h and 10.2 h).

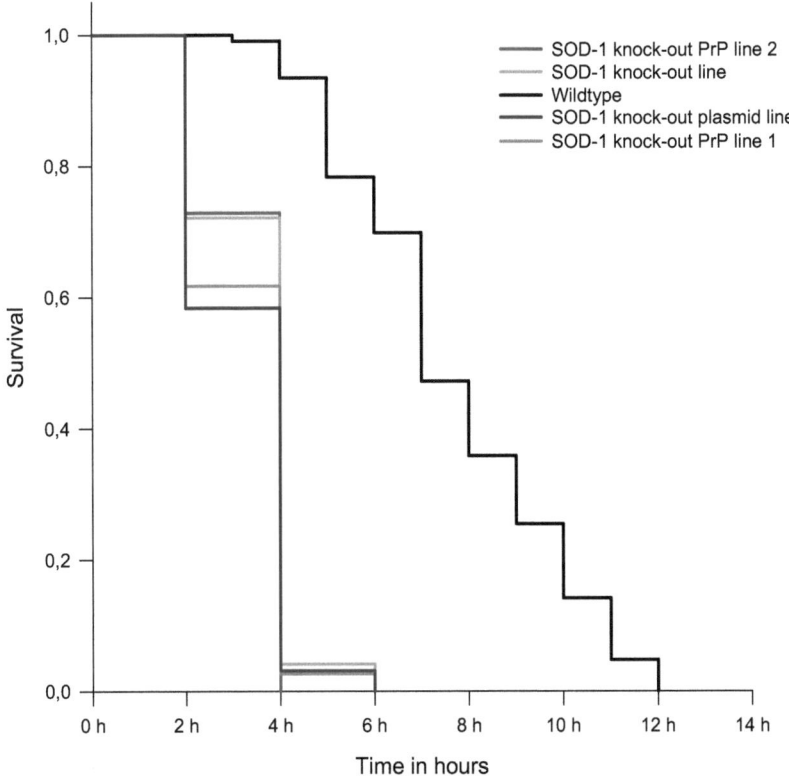

Figure 22: Lifespan under Paraquat of SOD-1 knock-out in PrP^C vs. no PrP^C expressing strains
Diagram showing wildtype (n = 106), SOD-1 knock-out PrP line 2 (n = 114) and SOD-1 knock-out PrP line 1 (n = 115), SOD-1 knock-out plasmid line (n = 197), and SOD-1 knock-out line (n = 147). There is no statistically significant difference between SOD-1 knock-out line and SOD-1 knock-out PrP line 1 (p = 0.0702; critical level = 0.0102), SOD-1 knock-out PrP line 2 (p = 0.563; critical level = 0.0253), SOD-1 knock-out plasmid line (p = 0.0123; critical level = 0.00730), between SOD-1 knock-out PrP line 1 and SOD-1 knock-out PrP line 2 (p = 0.197; critical level = 0.0170), SOD-1 knock-out plasmid line (p = 0.650; critical level = 0.0500), between SOD-1 knock-out PrP line 2 and SOD-1 knock-out plasmid line (p = 0.0637; critical level = 0.00851). There is a statistically significant difference between wildtype and SOD-1 knock-out line (p = 3.323E-44; critical level = 0.00366), SOD-1 knock-out PrP line 1 (p = 6.468E-42; critical level = 0.00394), ECSOD-1 knock-out plasmid line (p = 5.668E-51; critical level = 0.00341). Mean lifespan being 3.5 h for SOD-1 knock-out PrP line 2 (Std. = 0.08), 3.3 h for SOD-1 knock-out PrP line 1 (Std. = 0.1), 3.2 h for SOD-1 knock-out plasmid line (Std. = 0.08), 3.5 h for SOD-1 knock-out line (Std. = 0.8), 7.6 h for wildtype (Std. = 0.2).
Significance level = 0.05. Y-axis showing the relative population size; x-axis showing a time frame in hours.

Results

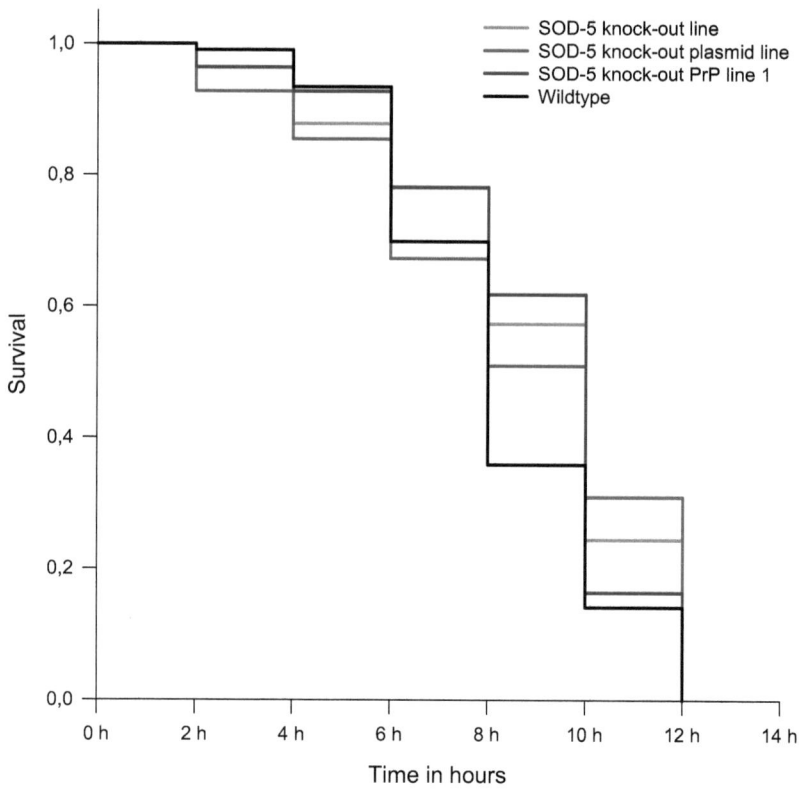

Figure 23: Lifespan under Paraquat of SOD-5 knock-out in PrP^C vs. no PrP^C expressing strains
Diagram showing wildtype (n = 106), SOD-5 knock-out plasmid line (n = 55), SOD-5 knock-out line (n = 82), SOD-5 knock-out PrP line 1 (n = 55). There is no statistically significant difference between wildtype and SOD-5 knock-out plasmid line (p = 0.0794; critical level = 0.0127), SOD-5 knock-out line (p = 0.0190; critical level = 0.00851), SOD-5 knock-out PrP line 1 (p = 0.0601; critical level = 0.0102), between SOD-5 knock-out plasmid line and SOD-5 knock-out line (p = 0.990; critical level = 0.0500), SOD-5 knock-out PrP line 1 (p = 0.0601; critical level = 0.0102), between SOD-5 knock-out line and SOD-5 knock-out PrP line 1 (p = 0.713; critical level = 0.0170). Mean lifespan being 8.2 h for wildtype (Std. = 0.2), 8.9 h for SOD-5 knock-out PrP line 1 (Std. = 0.3), 8.5 h for SOD-5 knock-out plasmid line (Std. = 0.4) and 8.8 h for SOD-5 knock-out line (Std. = 0.3).
Significance level = 0.05. Y-axis showing the relative population size; x-axis showing a time frame in hours.

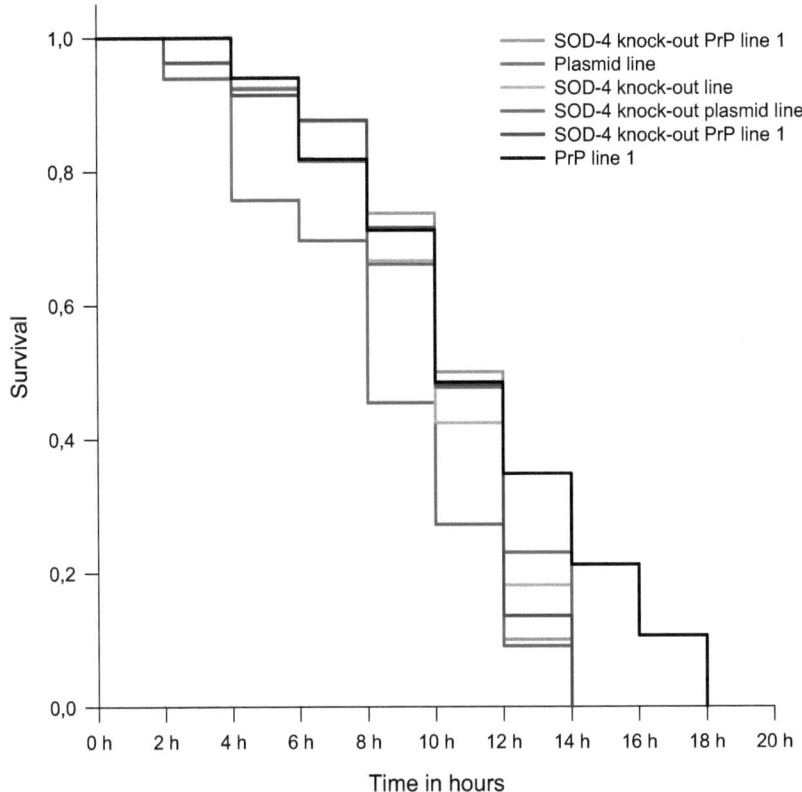

Figure 24: Lifespan under Paraquat of SOD-4 knock-out in PrP^C vs. no PrP^C expressing strains

Diagram showing plasmid line (n = 66), PrP line 1 (n = 66), SOD-4 knock-out PrP line 1 (n = 80) and SOD-4 knock-out PrP line 2 (n = 81), SOD-4 knock-out plasmid line (n = 65) and SOD-4 knock-out line (n = 66). There is no statistically significant difference between plasmid line and SOD-4 knock-out PrP line 1 (p = 0.00510; critical level = 0.00427), SOD-4 knock-out PrP line 2 (p = 0.00486; critical level = 0.00366), SOD-4 knock-out plasmid line (p = 0.00508; critical level = 0.00394), SOD-4 knock-out line (p = 0.0185; critical level = 0.00639), between PrP line 1 and SOD-4 knock-out PrP line 1 (p = 0.00935; critical level = 0.00568), SOD-4 knock-out PrP line 2 (p = 0.00886; critical level = 0.00512), SOD-4 knock-out plasmid line (p = 0.0229; critical level = 0.00730), SOD-4 knock-out line (p = 0.00829; critical level = 0.00465), between SOD-4 knock-out PrP line 1 and SOD-4 knock-out PrP line 2 (p = 0.896; critical level = 0.0253), SOD-4 knock-out plasmid line (p = 0.501; critical level = 0.00851), SOD-4 knock-out line (p = 0.959; critical level = 0.0500), between SOD-4 knock-out PrP line 2 and SOD-4 knock-out plasmid line (p = 0.599; critical level = 0.0127), SOD-4 knock-out line (p = 0.873; critical level = 0.0170), between SOD-4 knock-out plasmid line and SOD-4 knock-out line (p = 0.563; critical level = 0.0102). There is a statistically significant difference between plasmid line

and PrP line 1 (p = 0.0000183; critical level = 0.00341). Mean lifespan being 11.2 h (Std. = 0.5) for PrP line 1, 10.2 h (Std. = 0.3) for SOD-4 knock-out PrP line 2, 10.1 h (Std. = 0.4) for SOD-4 knock-out plasmid line, 9.9 h (Std. = 0.4) for SOD-4 knock-out line, 8.4 h (Std. = 0.4) for plasmid line, 10.2 h (Std. = 0.3) for SOD-4 knock-out PrP line 1.
Significance level = 0.05. Y-axis showing the relative population size; x-axis showing a time frame in hours.

3.4.5 Delta 8 deletion

The N-Terminal octarepeat region of PrP^C is rich in histidine, which, in turn, is responsible for a pH dependent binding of Cu^{2+}, and therefore of major dispute for its importance in possible functions of prion protein. In this trial, PrP^C was deleted from this region (residues 51-91), called delta 8 ($\Delta 8$), and compared to wildtype as well as to a natural PrP^C expressing line in a Paraquat stress scenario.

Figure 25 illustrates that there is no statistically significant difference between PrP^C expressing *C. elegans* line PrP line 1, PrP line 2 and $\Delta 8$. All three of them, however, show a statistically significant difference to wildtype or a significantly higher resistance to Paraquat (mean lifespan of 9.4 – 10.4 h compared to 7.9 h in wildtype).

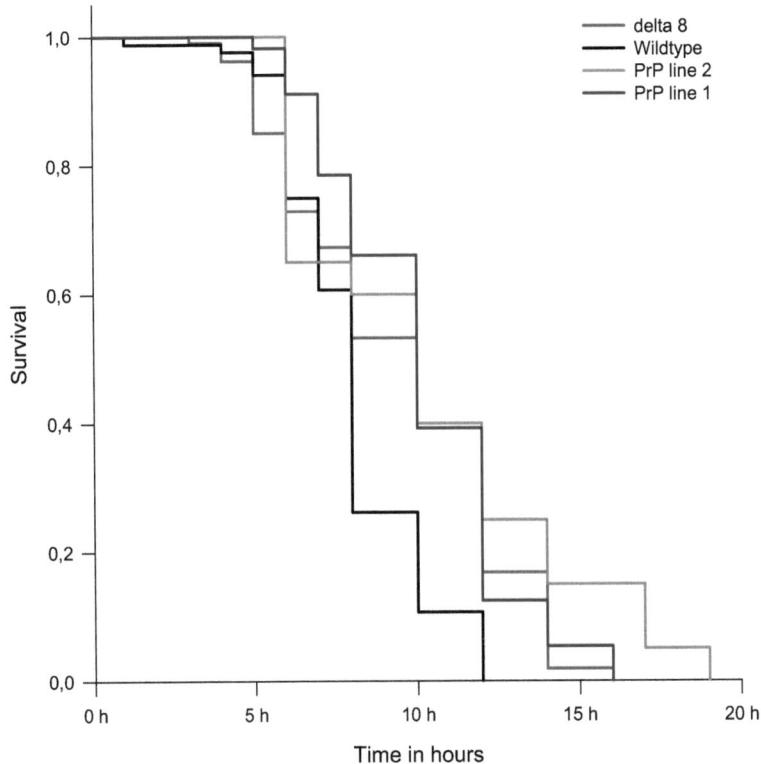

Figure 25: Lifespan under Paraquat in Δ8 vs. PrP^C expressing strain vs. wildtype
Diagram showing wildtype (n = 84), PrP line 1 (n = 56) and PrP line 2 (n = 20), Δ8 (n = 107). There is no statistically significant difference between PrP line 1 and PrP line 2 (p = 0.340; critical level = 0.0253), delta 8 (p = 0.450; critical level = 0.0500), between PrP line 2 and delta 8 (p = 0.125; critical level = 0.0170). There is a statistically significant difference between wildtype and PrP line 1 (p = 0.00000151; critical level = 0.00851), PrP line 2 (p = 0.00142; critical level = 0.0127) and delta 8 (p = 0.0000420; critical level = 0.0102). The mean lifespan is 10.1 h for PrP line 1 (Std. = 0.4), 10.4 h for PrP line 2 (Std. = 0.9), 7.9 h for wildtype (0.2) and 9.4 h for delta 8 (Std. = 0.3).
Significance level = 0.05. Y-axis showing the relative population size; x-axis showing a time frame in hours.

3.5 Heat stress assays

Heat being another common stressor in *C. elegans* used to investigate stress pathway mechanisms, in this trial, different *C. elegans* lines were stressed by 36 °C and their lifespan was concomitantly observed.

In figure 26, the behavior of lines expressing prion protein and those which do not were documented. The graph illustrates a very similar pattern between all lines and no statistically significant difference would likely be assumed. There is also no statistically significant difference between the lines except between plasmid line and PrP line 1, which are also the lines with the biggest difference in mean lifespan (8.6 h for PrP line 1 and 9.9 h for plasmid line).

The effects of DAF-16/FoxO knock-out can be surveyed in figure 27. Compared to wildtype, the DAF-16/FoxO knock-out lines all have a significant shorter lifespan pattern than wildtype. All DAF-16/FoxO lines, when compared to each other, are not in the statistically significant difference range, and show an almost identical lifespan pattern with their mean lifespan being between 5.9 h and 6.6 h.

Figure 28 compares wildtype with SOD-1 knock-out line. The different lines show a very similar lifespan behavior and also have no statistically significant difference, with their mean lifespan differing by just 0.1 h (8.8 h for SOD-1 knock-out line, 8.9 h for wildtype).

In the $\Delta 8$ line prion protein has been modified by a deletion of the N-terminal octarepeats (residues 51-91). In figure 29 this $\Delta 8$ *C. elegans* line was compared with PrP line 2 and plasmid line. On the graph all three seem to have a similar lifespan pattern when stressed by heat, and there is no statistically significant difference between PrP line 2 and plasmid line. There is one, however, between $\Delta 8$ and the other two with a slight elongated lifespan pattern for $\Delta 8$ (mean lifespan of 7.9 h for $\Delta 8$ compared to 7 h for PrP line 2 and 6.6 h for plasmid line).

Results

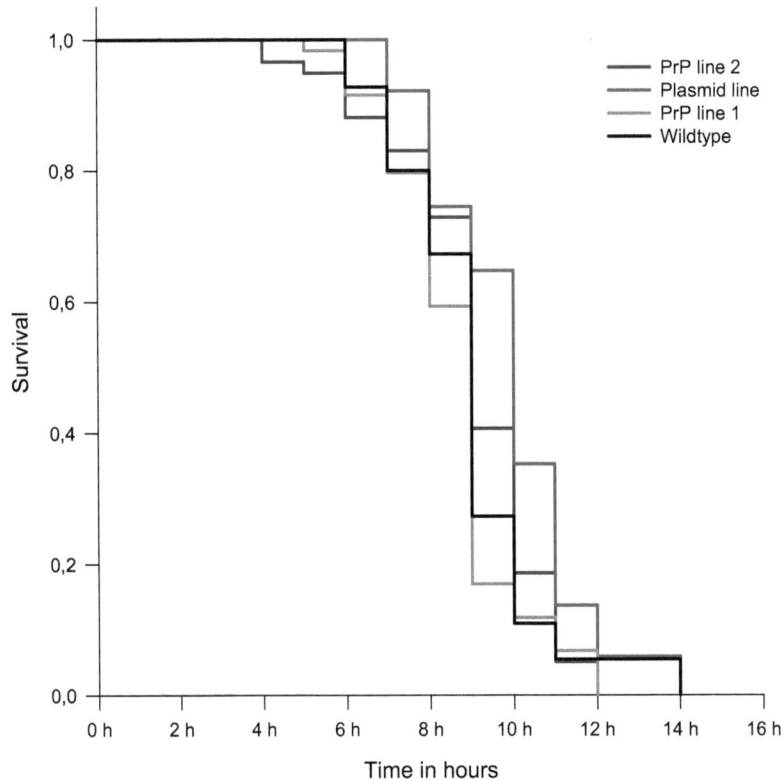

Figure 26: Lifespan under heat of PrP^C vs. no PrP^C expressing strains
Diagram showing wildtype (n = 55), plasmid line (n = 51), PrP line 1 (n = 59) and PrP line 2 (n = 59). There is no statistically significant difference between wildtype and plasmid line (p = 0.00454; critical level = 0.00366), PrP line 1 (p = 0.294; critical level = 0.00851), PrP line 2 (p = 0.510; critical level = 0.0127), between plasmid line and PrP line 2 (p = 0.0112; critical level = 0.00394), between PrP line 1 and PrP line 2 (p = 0.123; critical level = 0.00512). There is a statistically significant difference between plasmid line and PrP line 1 (p = 0.000225; critical level = 0.00320). The mean lifespan being 8.9 h for wildtype (Std. = 0.2), 8.6 h for PrP line 1 (Std. = 0.2), 9.9 h for plasmid line (Std. = 0.2), 9.0 h for PrP line 2 (Std. = 0.2).
Significance level = 0.05. Y-axis showing the relative population size; x-axis showing a time frame in hours.

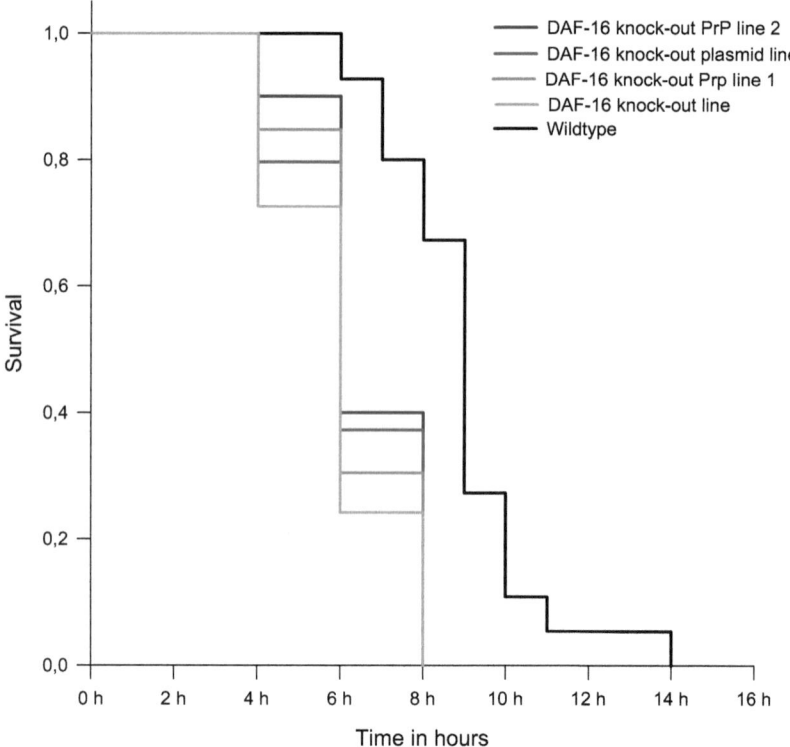

Figure 27: Lifespan under heat of DAF-16/FoxO knock-out in PrP^C vs. no PrP^C expressing strains
DAF-16/FoxO, Abnormal dauer formation / Forkhead transcription factor; PrP^C, Cellular protease resistant protein. Diagram showing wildtype (n = 55), DAF-16 knock-out line (n = 62), DAF-16 knock-out plasmid line (n = 59), DAF-16 knock-out PrP line 2 (n = 60) and DAF-16 knock-out PrP line 1 (n = 59). There is no statistically significant difference between DAF-16 knock-out line and DAF-16 knock-out plasmid line (p = 0.117; critical level = 0.00465), DAF-16 knock-out PrP line 2 (p = 0.0136; critical level = 0.00427), DAF-16 knock-out PrP line 1 (p = 0.185; critical level = 0.00568), between DAF-16 knock-out plasmid line and DAF-16 knock-out PrP line 2 (p = 0.436; critical level = 0.0102) DAF-16 knock-out PrP line 1 (p = 0,727; critical level 0.0170), DAF-16 knock-out PrP line 2 and DAF-16 knock-out PrP line 1 (p = 0.226; critical level = 0.00730). There is a statistically significant difference between wildtype and DAF-16 knock-out line (p = 2,937E-17; critical level = 0.00165), DAF-16 knock-out plasmid line (p = 1.482E-14; critical level = 0.00213), DAF-16 knock-out PrP line 2 (p = 4.365E-14; critical level = 0.00233); DAF-16 knock-out PrP line 1 (p = 1.417E-15; critical level = 0.00190). The mean lifespan being 5.9 h for DAF-16 knock-out line (Std. = 0.2), 6.3 h for DAF-16 knock-out PrP line 1 (Std. = 0.2), 6.3 h for DAF-16 knock-out plasmid line (Std. = 0.2), 6.6 h for DAF-16 knock-out PrP line 2 (Std. = 0.2), 8.9 h for wildtype (Std. = 0.2).
Significance level = 0.05. Y-axis showing the relative population size; x-axis showing a time frame in hours.

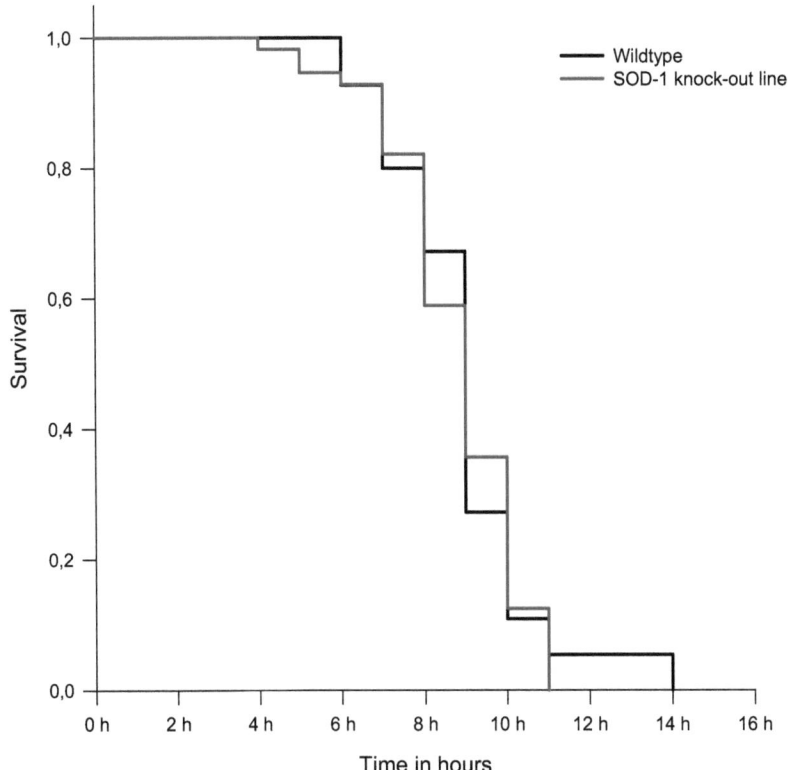

Figure 28: **Lifespan under heat of SOD-1 knock-out vs. wildtype**
Diagram showing wildtype (n = 55) and SOD-1 knock-out line (n = 56). There is no statistically significant difference between wildtype and SOD-1 knock-out line (p = 0.841; critical level = 0.0500). The mean lifespan being 8.9 h for wildtype (Std. = 0.2) and 8.8 h for SOD-1 knock-out line (Std. = 0.2).
Significance level = 0.05. Y-axis showing the relative population size; x-axis showing a time frame in hours.

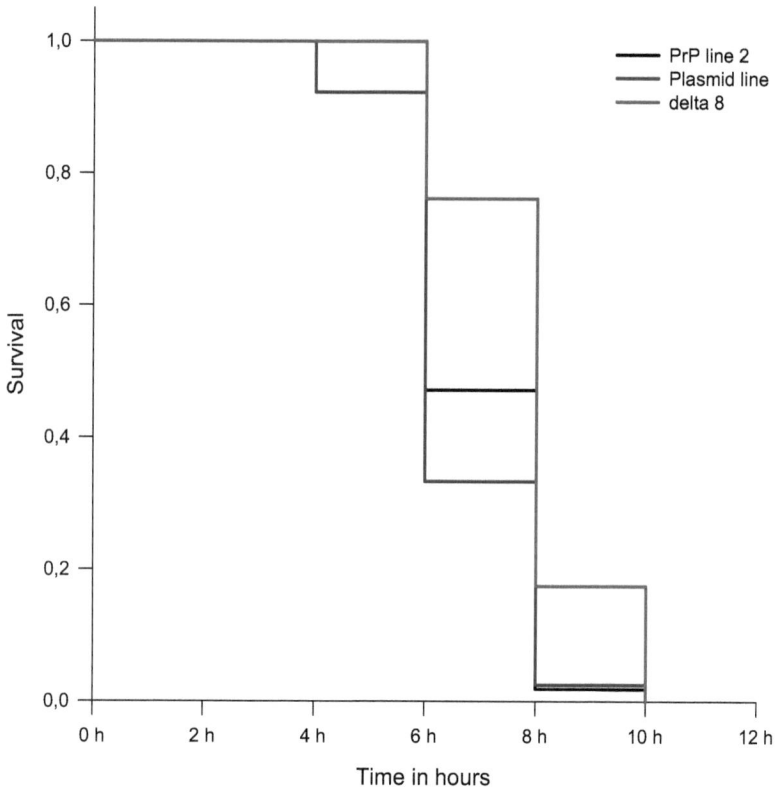

Figure 29: Lifespan under heat of Δ8 prion protein vs. PrP^C expressing strains
Diagram showing plasmid line (n = 39), PrP line 2 (n = 53) and Δ8 (n = 63). There is no statistically significant difference between plasmid line and PrP line 2 (p = 0.137; critical level = 0.0170). There is a statistically significant difference between plasmid line and delta 8 (p = 6.620E-6; critical level = 0.00427), between PrP line 2 and delta 8 (p = 0.000140; critical level = 0.00512). The mean lifespan being 7.9 h for delta 8 (Std. = 0.2), 6.6 h for plasmid line (Std. = 0.2) and 7.0 h for PrP line 2 (Std. = 0.1).
Significance level = 0.05. Y-axis showing the relative population size; x-axis showing a time frame in hours.

3.6 Copper stress assay

Cu^{2+} ions, on one hand, play an essential part in detoxification of oxidative stress, as in the case of superoxide dismutase. On the other hand, it can cause oxidative stress or toxicity on its own if its concentration exceeds physiological standards. In this lifespan experiment, a concentration of 0.8 mM Cu^{2+}, achieved by a $CuSO_4$ solution, was chosen to determine the behavior of *C. elegans* to this stressor. In this case no prion protein expressing lines (wildtype and plasmid line) were compared to prion protein expressing lines (PrP line 1 and PrP line 2).

Figure 30, on the one hand, illustrates the whole lifespan of those four lines under copper stress, while, on the other hand, the grey dotted line sets an imaginative border at 156 h (6.5 days), meaning that all worms still alive at that point were counted dead at the point of 156 h.

Observing the lifespan curves, it can be seen that all four lines show an almost identical lifespan behavior until the above mentioned 156 h point, which includes 98.5% of the wildtype worms and 92.8% of its maximum lifespan, while, in contrast, 80.0% of the PrP line 1 worms and 72.2% of its maximum lifespan, and the plasmid line and PrP line 2 lie in between. The lines spread after the point of 156 h, with PrP line 1 being the most resistant (mean lifespan = 141.7 h) and wildtype the least (mean lifespan = 133 h). Plasmid line and PrP line 2 were almost identical in the middle, leading to statistically significant differences between wildtype, plasmid line, and PrP line 1, as well as between PrP line 1 and PrP line 2. This was not the case for the other matches.

If this "end-point-spread" of the lines is ignored by taking the grey dotted 156 h limit, then no statistically significant difference can be found, with the mean lifespan of all lines ranging between 131.8 h (PrP line 1) and 135.6 h (plasmid line).

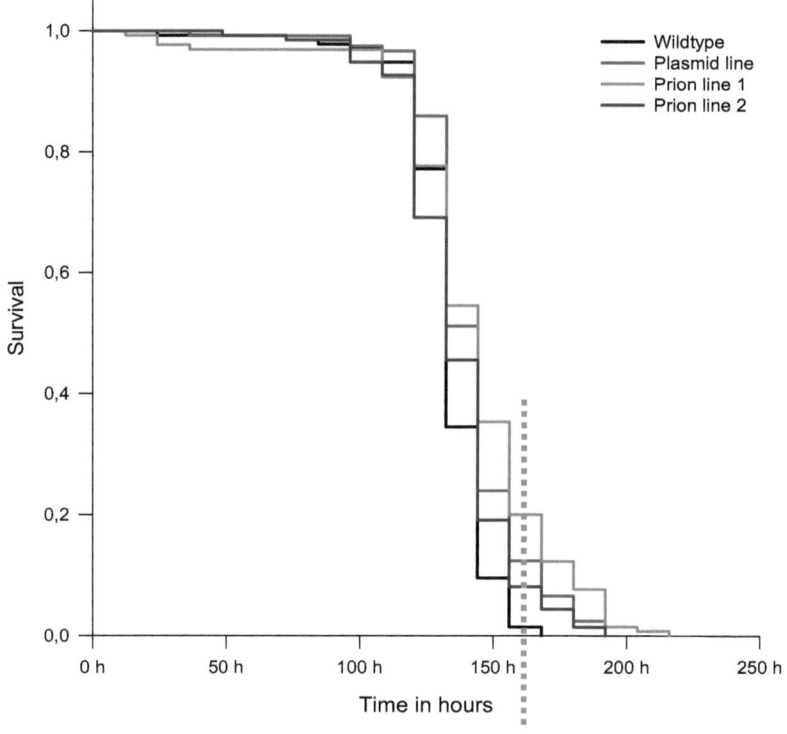

Figure 30: Lifespan under Cu^{2+} of PrP^C vs. no PrP^C expressing strains

Diagram showing wildtype (n = 136), plasmid line (n = 121), PrP line 1 (n = 130) and PrP line 2 (n = 136). There is no statistically significant difference between wildtype and PrP line 2 (p = 0.0509; critical value = 0.0170), between plasmid line and PrP line 2 (p = 0.0735; critical value = 0.0253); PrP line 1 (p = 0.137; critical value = 0.0500). There is a statistically significant difference between wildtype and PrP line 1 (p = 1.350E-6; critical level = 0.00851), plasmid line (p = 0.0000647; critical level = 0.0102), between PrP line 1 and PrP line 2 (p = 0.00206; critical level = 0.0127). Mean lifespan being 135.7 h for PrP line 2 (Std. = 1.8), 141.7 h for PrP line 1 (Std. = 2.7), 140.8 h for plasmid line (Std. = 1.8) and 133.0 h for wildtype (Std. = 1.4).

Considering the 156 h limit: There is no statistically significant difference between wildtype and plasmid line (p = 0.0557; critical level = 0.00851), PrP line 1 (p = 0.123; critical level = 0.0102), PrP line 2 (p = 0.703 ; critical level = 0.0253), between

plasmid line and PrP line 1 (p = 0.925; critical level = 0.0500), PrP line 2 (p = 0.187; critical level = 0.0127), between PrP line 1 and PrP line 2 (p = 0.267; critical level = 0.0170). The mean lifespan being 132.1 h for PrP line 2 (Std. = 1.6), 131.8 h for PrP line 1 (Std. = 2.5), 135.6 h for plasmid line (Std. = 1.5) and 132.4 h for wildtype (Std. = 1.4).

Significance level = 0.05. Y-axis showing the relative population size; x-axis showing a time frame in hours.

3.7 Paraquat stress assay after previous Cu^{2+} treatment

Paraquat is a creator of $O_2^{\cdot-}$ superoxide anions, which become detoxified in the organism by various SODs, which, in turn, SOD1, 4, and 5 use Cu^{2+} as a biocatalyst. PrP^C does contain a histidine rich region (residues 51-91) which is able to bind Cu^{2+}. Therefore, it was to the intention of this trial to observe if the expression of prion protein has either positive or negative influences on the resistance of *C. elegans* towards Paraquat compared to those which do not express PrP^C if treated with an non-lethal concentration of 0.2 mM Cu^{2+} beforehand.

Figure 31 shows the result of this trial in the form of the copper treated lines wildtype Cu^{2+}, plasmid line Cu^{2+} and PrP line 2 Cu^{2+}, as well as plasmid line as a control which had not previously been treated with Cu^{2+}. The survival behavior of the *C. elegans* lines is diffuse with statistical significant differences between all lines except between plasmid line and plasmid line Cu^{2+}. Observing the graph, it seems wildtype Cu^{2+} and PrP line 2 Cu^{2+} have a decreased Paraquat resistance compared to plasmid line control and plasmid line Cu^{2+}.

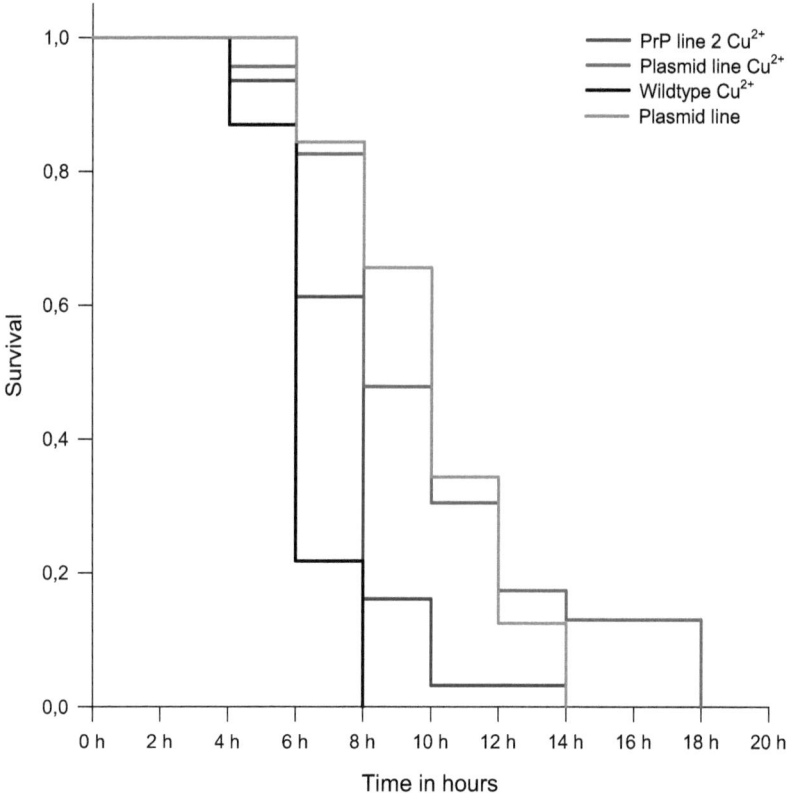

Figure 31: Lifespan under previous Cu2+ loading of PrP^C vs. no PrP^C expressing strains
Diagram showing copper treated wildtype Cu$^{2=}$ (n = 23), copper treated plasmid line Cu^{2+} (n = 23), copper treated PrP line 2 Cu^{2+} (n = 31) and plasmid line (n = 32). There is a statistically significant difference between wildtype Cu$^{2=}$ and plasmid line control (p = 1.090E-8; critical level = 0.00851), plasmid line Cu^{2+} (p = 0.00000566; critical level = 0.0102), PrP line 2 Cu$^{2=}$ (0.00227; critical level = 0.0170), between PrP line 2 Cu$^{2=}$ and plasmid line Cu^{2+} (p = 0.00376; critical level = 0.0253), plasmid line control (p = 0.000150; critical level = 0.0127). There is no statistically significant difference between plasmid line Cu^{2+} and plasmid line control (p = 0.813; critical level = 0.0500). The mean lifespan being 6.2 h for wildtype Cu^{2+} (Std. = 0.2), 10 h for plasmid line Cu^{2+} (Std. = 0.8), 7.5 h for PrP line 2 Cu^{2+} (Std. = 0.4), 9.9 h for plasmid line control (Std. = 0.4).
Significance level = 0.05. Y-axis showing the relative population size; x-axis showing a time frame in hours.

3.8 Hydrogen peroxide stress assay

Hydrogen peroxide (H_2O_2) is the outcome of the detoxification process of $O_2^{\cdot-}$ by SODs, but is also another reactive oxidant species (ROS) which requires further breakdown by substances such as glutathione or catalase. In this lifespan experiment it was the intention to observe differences in *C. elegans* handling H_2O_2 in respect to expressing prion protein as opposed to having a SOD-1 knock-out.

Figure 32 illustrates several *C. elegans* lines which were continuously exposed to 1.7 mM H_2O_2. To all appearances, PrP line 1 and control lines (plasmid line, wildtype) seem to have a very similar survival pattern, while PrP line 2 and SOD-1 knock-out line show a slight decreased resistance, although only being statistically significant for SOD-1 knock-out line. This is also expressed in the statistics with no significant difference between PrP line 2, PrP line 1 and wildtype except between PrP line 2 and plasmid line, or with significant differences between SOD-1 knock-out line and the others, with the exception of PrP line 2. DAF-16/FoxO knock-out lines, on the other hand, have an almost identical survival pattern in comparison with each other, with no statistically significant differences but show a statistically as well as visibly significant reduction in lifespan compared to the rest.

In Figure 33, a different approach is illustrated. Instead of exposing nematodes continuously to the alleged toxin, worms were shock exposed to 2 mM of H_2O_2 for 45 min and then placed on regular plates for observation. As all lines reached a stable survival level after 12 h at the latest, the experiment was therefore terminated after 24 h. Here, prion protein lines (PrP line 2, PrP line 1) seem to have a reduced survival pattern compared to control lines (plasmid line, wildtype), but this is only expressed with a statistically significant difference between PrP line 2 and plasmid line or wildtype, but not for PrP line 1, which has an almost identical behavior in the first 8 hours, but then has a higher base line population than PrP line 2. This makes it not significantly different from wildtype and plasmid line. SOD-1 knock-out line, on the other hand, is characterized by a very steep drop in survival at the 6th hour, which is expressed in statistically significant differences to wildtype and plasmid line, but not to PrP line 1 and PrP line 2.

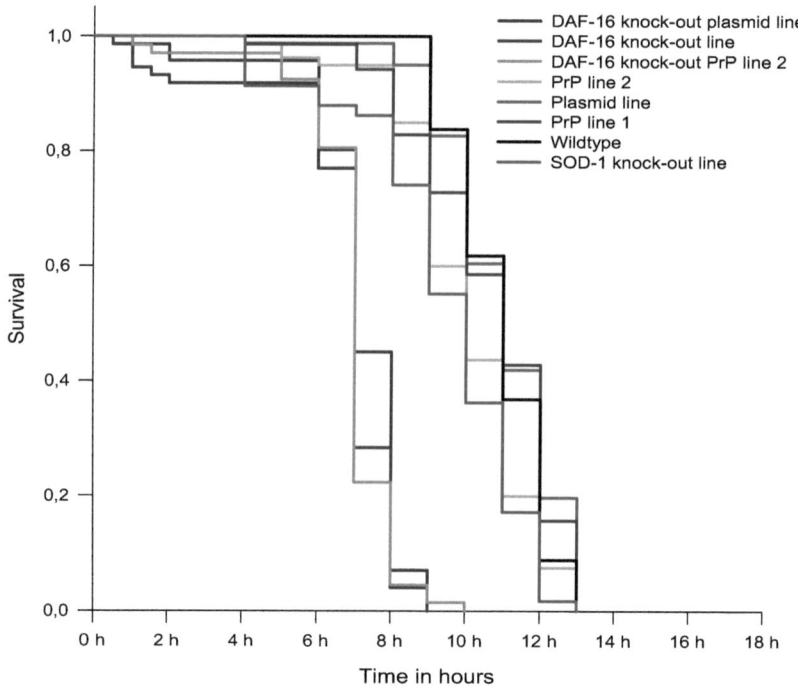

Figure 32: Lifespan under continuous 1.7 mM H$_2$O$_2$ exposure

Diagram showing wildtype (n = 68), plasmid line (n = 81), PrP line 2 (n = 80) and PrP line 1 (n = 70), SOD-1 knock-out line (n = 58), DAF-16 knock-out line (n = 74), DAF-16 knock-out plasmid line (n = 71), DAF-16 knock-out PrP line 2 (n = 67). There is no statistically significant difference between wildtype and PrP line 2 (p = 0.0109; critical level = 0.00568), plasmid line (p = 0.296; critical level = 0.0127), PrP line 1 (p = 0.714; critical level = 0.0253), between PrP line 1 and PrP line 2 (p = 0.0143; critical level = 0.00639) and plasmid line (p = 0.499; critical level = 0.0170), between DAF-16 knock-out line and DAF-16 knock-out plasmid line (p = 0.0718; critical level = 0.00730), DAF-16 knock-out PrP line 2 (p = 0.970; critical level = 0.0500), between DAF-16 knock-out plasmid line and DAF-16 knock-out PrP line 2 (p = 0.0733; critical level = 0.00851). There is a statistically significant difference between DAF-16 knock-out line and plasmid line (p = 1.211E-34; critical level = 0.00183), wildtype (p = 3.207E-33; critical level = 0.00190), PrP line 2 (p = 6.324E-27; critical level = 0.00233), PrP line 1 (p = 4.695E-26; critical level = 0.00244), SOD-1 knock-out line (p = 1.159E-16; critical level = 0.00320), between DAF-16 knock-out PrP line 2 and plasmid line (p = 5.271E-33; critical level = 0.00197), wildtype (p = 8.649E-32; critical level = 0.00213), PrP line 2 (p = 1.686E-025; critical level = 0.00256), PrP line 1 (p = 3.306E-25; critical level = 0.00270), SOD-1 knock-out line (p = 1.449E-15; critical level = 0.00341), between DAF-16 knock-out plasmid line and plasmid line (p = 1.022E-32; critical level = 0.00205), wildtype (p = 1.471E-31; critical level = 0.00223), PrP line 2 (p = 2.625E-24; critical level = 0.00285), PrP line 1 (p = 1.019E-23; critical level = 0.00301), SOD-1 knock-out line (p = 7.739E-15; critical level = 0.00366), between SOD-1 knock-out line and plasmid line (p = 0.0000128; critical level = 0.00394), wildtype (p = 0.000200; critical level = 0.00427), PrP line 1 (p = 0.000450; critical level = 0.00465), between plasmid line and PrP line 2 (p = 0.000842; critical level = 0.00512). The mean lifespan being 9.4 h for SOD-1 knock-out line (Std. = 0.3), 10.9 h for wildtype (Std. = 0.1), 10.6 h for PrP line 1 (Std. = 0.2), 11.0 h for plasmid line (Std. = 0.2), 10.0 h for PrP line 2 (Std. = 0.2), 6.9 h for DAF-16 knock-out PrP line 2 (Std. = 0.2), 6.7 h for DAF-16 knock-out line (Std. = 0.2) and 7.1 h for DAF-16 knock-out plasmid line (Std. = 0.2). Significance level = 0.05. Y-axis showing the relative population size; x-axis showing a time frame in hours.

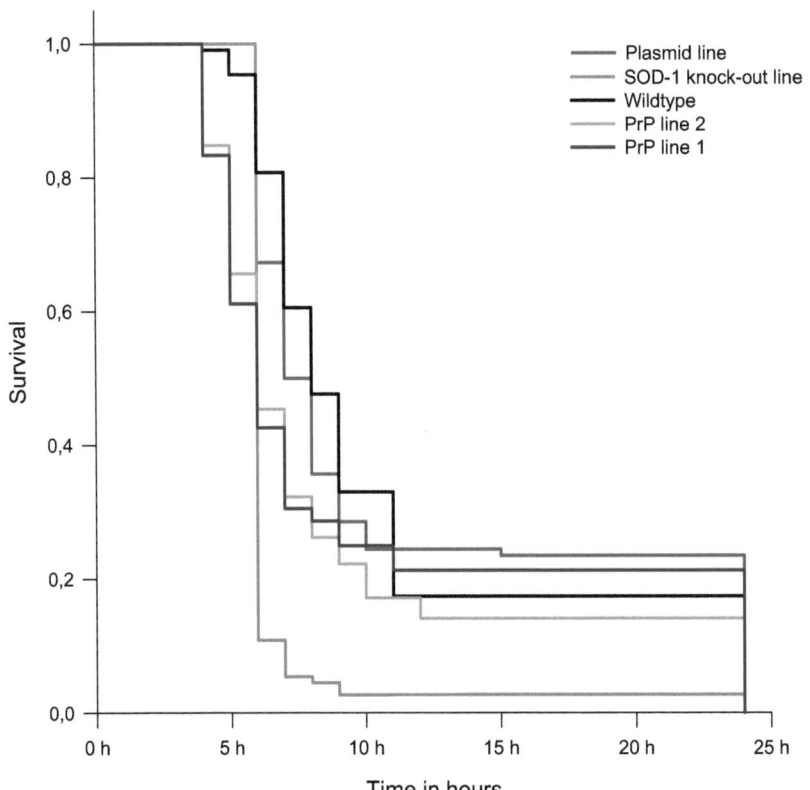

Figure 33: Lifespan after 45 min of 2 mM peroxide exposure of PrPC, no PrPC and SOD-1 knock-out expressing strains

Diagram showing wildtype (n = 109), plasmid line (n = 98), PrP line 2 (n = 99) and PrP line 1 (n = 108), SOD-1 knock-out line (n = 110). There is no statistically significant difference between PrP line 1 and plasmid line (p = 0.00842; critical level = 0.00639), wildtype (p = 0.00902; critical level = 0.00730), SOD-1 knock-out line (p = 0.255; critical level = 0.0102), PrP line 2 (p = 0.589; critical level = 0.0170), between SOD-1 knock-out line and PrP line 2 (p = 0.126; critical level = 0.00851), between wildtype and plasmid line (p = 0.676; critical

level = 0.0500). There is a statistically significant difference between SOD-1 knock-out line and wildtype (p = 2.790E-18; critical level = 0.00341), plasmid line (p = 1.210E-14; critical level = 0.00366), between PrP line 2 and wildtype (p = 0.000562; critical level = 0.00512), plasmid line (p = 0.00135; critical level = 0.00568). The mean lifespan being 9.7 h for PrP line 1 (Std. = 0.7), 8.8 h for PrP line 2 (Std. = 0.7), 10.8 h for wildtype (Std. = 0.6), 6.6 h for SOD-1 knock-out line (Std. = 0.3) and 11.2 h for plasmid line (Std. = 0.7).
Significance level = 0.05. Y-axis showing the relative population size; x-axis showing a time frame in hours.

3.9 SOD enzyme assay

Unlike in the human being, *C. elegans* expresses five instead of three SODs, of which two are MnSODs (SOD-2, SOD-3) with three Cu/ZnSODs (SOD-1, SOD-4, SOD-5). This trial attempted to inhibit, with an SOD Enzyme Assay either MnSODs by a mix of ethanol and chloroform, or Cu/ZnSODs by KCN, to contrast a possible difference in expression or activity of SODs, between prion protein expressing PrP line 2 and PrP line 1, prion protein non-expressing plasmid line and SOD-1 knock-out SOD-1 knock-out line.

In figure 34, the different activity levels of all SODs (untreated), ethanol or cyanide inhibited SODs of the different *C. elegans* lines are illustrated in units per microgram under unstressed conditions. PrP line 2 and plasmid line rely on a similar ratio of Cu/ZnSODs to MnSODs while PrP line 1, on the other hand, shows a different ratio which relies more on Cu/ZnSODs. PrP line 1 also presents with nearly double the overall SOD activity than PrP line 2 and plasmid line. OH 7600 shows that SOD-1 accounts for the majority of Cu/ZnSODs, since, under ethanol inhibition, almost no activity is left compared to the other strains.

Figure 35 shows the different SOD activity levels in the same fashion as in figure 34 but under Paraquat stress conditions. In this case a switch in SOD activities is visible. While plasmid line does not really change its SOD profile under stress compared to no stress, PrP line 2 clearly focuses on Cu/ZnSODs, which now looks like the SOD profile PrP line 1 had right from the start in figure 35. SOD-1 knock-out line, on the other hand, totally shuts down its SOD activity, thus showing that a lack of SOD-1 leads to a total SOD activity loss under Paraquat stress. Another phenomenon seen is the severe decline in overall SOD activity in all lines under stress compared to those in figure 35 of no stress.

Results

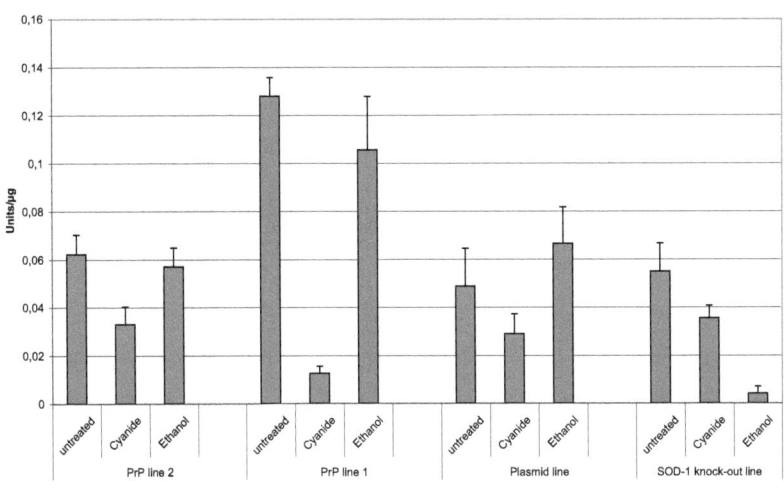

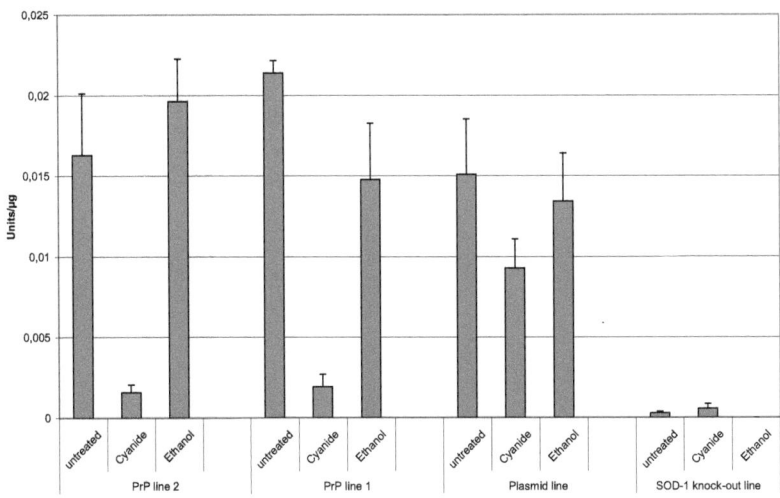

Figure 34 & 35: SOD Enzyme Activity Assay under "natural" conditions & SOD Enzyme Activity Assay after previous Paraquat exposure

Showing PrP line 2, PrP line 1, plasmid line and SOD-1 knock-out line. In all cases the amount n = undefined (= reaching several thousands). Each line is illustrated in three columns on the x-axis, untreated meaning all SODs are measured, cyanide meaning Cu/ZnSODs are inhibited, ethanol meaning MnSODs are inhibited. The y-axis naming the SOD activity in units/µg. The standard deviation is illustrated for each column. The activities were calculated by three trials with four values each. Figure 34 showing *C. elegans* in unstressed conditions, while Figure 35 showing lines under Paraquat stress.

3.10 Dye fill

Dye filling is a technique to stain amphid and phasmid neurons, which are accumulated in the head and tail of the nematode. In this context, the staining was used to compare the neurological uptake of dye in all *C. elegans* strains, and thereby illustrate inoculation differences between PrP^C expressing lines and lines not expression prion protein.

In figures 36-38 PrP line 1, plasmid line and wildtype are illustrated. PrP line 1 in both cases shows a whole nematode which has a fluorescenting line through its body with an accumulation or fluorescence cluster, respectively, at its head and a smaller one at its tail. Both clusters represent the amphid and phasmid neurons. The line in between shows its digestive tract.

Plasmid-carrying plasmid line only shows a head on the upper row and then a folded complete nematode at the lower row. At the upper one the clustered fluorescenting head neurons are clearly visible; the lower one shows the fluorescenting head and tail neurons. The digestive tract is not seen here, since in this case the dye has already passed the tract.

Only the heads are seen in wildtype *C. elegans*. In both cases bright fluorescence clustered in head neurons is visible. The digestive tract, however, is not visible, as the dye has already passed the tract.

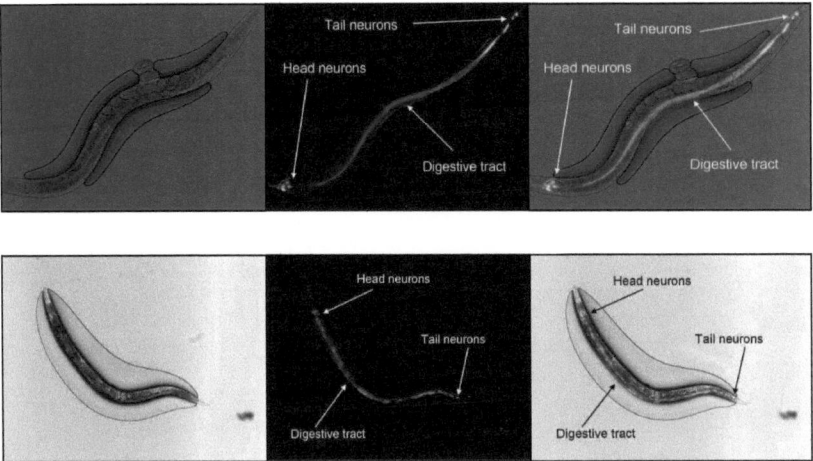

Figure 36: Dye Fill in PrP^C expressing strains

Both rows show a worm of PrP line 1 magnified by 200x each. The upper one is a young adult; head is at the lower left. Head neurons and digestive tract are clearly illuminated, tail neurons at the right far end, too. Lower row showing a L4 stage; head is at the upper left; again head as well as tail neurons and digestive tract are clearly visible by fluorescence.

Left images are visualized with a standard filter, middle ones with a Texas red filter, right ones show left and middle images digitally stacked on top of each other. Illumination time was at 40 ms.

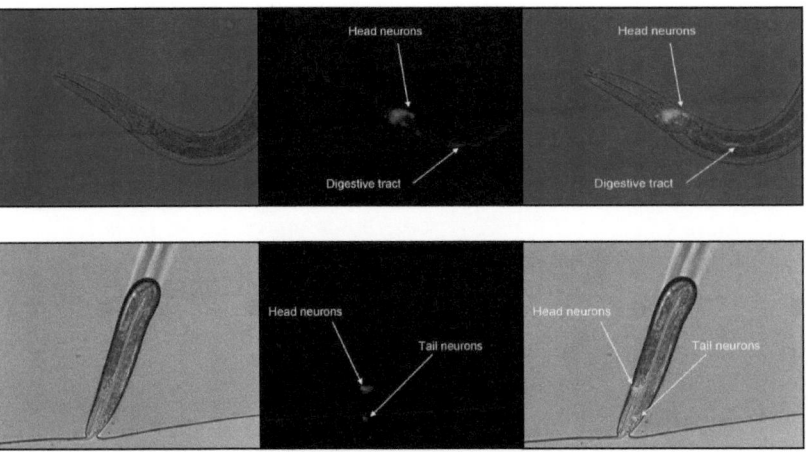

Results

Figure 37: Dye Fill in empty-plasmid strains
Both rows show a worm of plasmid line magnified by 400x.upper and 200x lower one. The upper one shows the head of an adult. Head neurons and beginning of the digestive tract are clearly illuminated. Lower row showing a folded young adult; head is at the left; head and tail neurons are clearly visible by fluorescence.
Left images are visualized with a standard filter, middle ones with a Texas red filter, right ones show left and middle images digitally stacked on top of each other. Illumination time was at 40 ms.

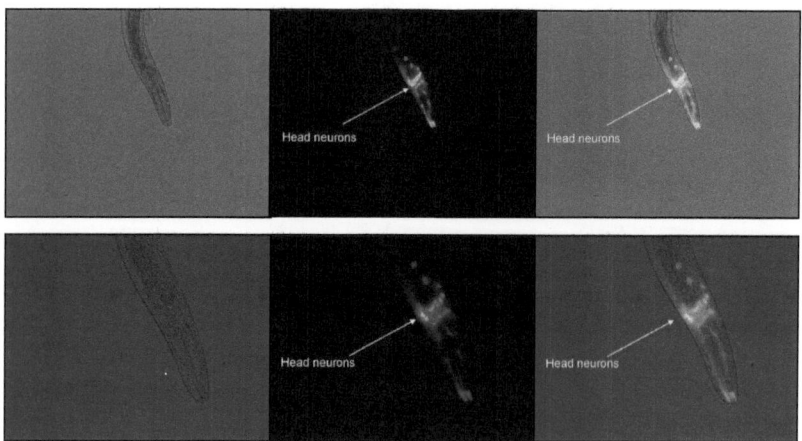

Figure 38: Dye Fill in wildtype
Both rows show the head region of wildtype magnified by 200x upper one and 400x lower one. The upper one shows the head of an L4. Head neurons are clearly illuminated. Lower row showing an adult; head neurons are clearly visible by fluorescence.
Left images are visualized with a standard filter, middle ones with a Texas red filter, right ones show left and middle images digitally stacked on top of each other. Illumination time was at 40 ms.

4 Discussion

4.1 Verification of the obtained data

4.1.1 Western blot

Some of the data shown (3.1 - 3.2) was collected to support or verify the primary data discussed in 4.2 - 4.3. Western blotting served the simple purpose of showing the expression and what exactly is expressed of PrP^C in the supposed strains over time, and thus samples were taken at several points. Since the protocol itself was done by long established standard procedure [37, 189], I am going to resign to discuss methodical aspects. PrP^C has its full molecular weight at around 38 kDa, however Western blot images reveal several PrP^C associated bands in strains expressing prion protein starting at around 22 kDa. The third band from the top is already identified by recPrP, which marks the unglycolysated PrP^C ($cytPrP^C$) at around 28 kDa [81, 132, 164]. The two bands on top with the higher molecular weight most likely represent mono- and diglyoclysated fragments of PrP^C. Usually prion protein is glycolysated at amino acids 181-183 and 197-199, therefore having a molecular weight of around 33-34 kDa if monoglycolysated or 38 kDa if diglycolysated [164]. However, these two bands range between 29 and 35 kDa, thus either representing glycolysated fragments of PrP^C or full-length PrP^C with smaller glycolysations. The bands underneath the unglycolysated one with a lower molecular weight are most likely different fragments of prion protein resulting from a failed complete inhibition of proteases. Although this phenomenon is not explicitly described in corresponding literature, a similar molecular weight distribution of PrP^C is seen by Glatzel and Aguzzi (2000) [74] and Lau et al. (2007) [113], especially if Proteinase K was added to characterize between PrP^C and PrP^{Sc}. Furthermore, analogue results are seen in studies investigating specific C1 and C2 cleavage fragments in which PrP^C is cleaved at residue 110 for C1 and at 90 for C2 producing C- and N- terminal fragments [45, 196]. Thus it can be assumed that PrP^C expression in *C. elegans* is successful, and resembles prion protein expression in already established model systems. However there are still many open questions which need to be answered in further research.

Discussion

4.1.2 GFP fluorescence

During this project we also applied the method of GFP fluorescence to achieve a verification of the data obtained. In our scenario we used GFP in two ways (3.1). In the first case GFP was inserted on an additional plasmid with the other two plasmids containing *Prnp* and *pha-1* which allowed us to conclude that inheritance of the plasmids and its translation is most likely to be successful if a GFP signal is obtained (figure 4). A second GFP was inserted in the SmaI-site of *Prnp* coding sequence [184] so that the localization of PrP^C in the nematode could have been documented (figure 5). Since we were able to express full length PrP^C in *C. elegans* for the first time, we have no literature and data to compare it to. However, the pictures illustrate that PrP^C is expressed in diverse membranic structures which we were not able to further characterize. Most likely these structures represent the endoplasmatic reticulum, or possibly extracellular membranes, suggesting a correct extracellular placement. [119, 168, 213, 222, 237]. Further research is essential to gaining a better knowledge about trafficking and expression patterns of huPrP^C in *C. elegans*.

4.1.3 Heat tolerance and pha-1

As the loss rate of the injected plasmids is high, a guarantee of successful prion protein inheritance through the use of a visual system such as GFP would have been very laborious, as an individual verification of every worm would have been necessary. Therefore, a more mass-implementation suitable system was used. For transgenic strains, a line with a temperature selective embryonic lethal mutation *pha-1 (e2323)* was taken as a basis. This caused the worm to grow normally at 15 °C. However, at 25 °C, the *pha-1* mutation is 100% embryonic lethal, as *pha-1* is essential for the thermosensitive midembryogenesis [176]. Thus, transgenic lines were dependent on the plasmid with the coinjected correct *pha-1* gene to survive and reproduce at 25 °C [75]. Therefore, every surviving transgenic worm has been one which was able to successfully express the plasmid products.

4.2 PrP^C involved in oxidative stress response

The objective of this work (1.4) was to illuminate the possible functions of PrP^C, which remains a hotly debated mystery. During my introduction, a diverse spectrum of proposed and controversially debated hypothesises about the physiological function of PrP^C were addressed (1.2.3 - 1.2.6), which, despite having no demand for completeness, gave an idea of how broad the possible functions of prion protein are, forcing one to focus on a specific spectrum from the beginning. I

Discussion

chose to do so by narrowinging in on the involvement of PrP^C in management of oxidative stress or reactive oxygen species (ROS).

4.2.1 Paraquat

To illustrate possible functions of PrP^C in processing of ROS or environmental stress, various approaches were chosen. The most acknowledged theories, mostly published by Brown, which regarded prion protein and ROS processing focused on the connection between PrP^C and the increase of an organism's SOD activity, more precisely SOD-1 [27, 33, 107, 170], or with PrP^C mimicking an SOD activity itself [27, 34]. This also has been challenged by partly opposing results such as those from Jones, who was not able to detect any SOD like activity above normal in a prion protein isolated medium [102], which is similar to Hutter and Waggoner, who both deny any connection of PrP^C to superoxide dismutase [92, 216]. This discussion continues most recently with La Mendola publishing that avian PrP^C does not does not have an SOD like activity, but mammalian PrP^C does *in vitro* [111], while Gaggelli sees only a faint activity in prion protein of zebrafishes, [70] and Sakudo fails to recognize any in GPI anchorless PrP^C [171].

4.2.1.1 PrP^C expressing vs. non-expressing strains

Consequently, a well established stressor of *C. elegans*, i.e. Paraquat, was chosen to bring more light into this hot topic [11, 69, 199]. Paraquat being a known producer of $O_2^{\cdot-}$ (1.2.5), we saw a significantly increased resistance of lines expressing PrP^C in Paraquat stress assays (3.4.1), with a later onset in dying and weaker decline in population size. As there is only one way to process $O_2^{\cdot-}$, namely by the conversion of superoxide ions into hydrogen peroxide by superoxide dismutase, it can be assumed that either an activation of the intracellular SOD-1 and/or SOD-5 of *C. elegans* [59, 230] by PrP^C is the reason, or that possibly an SOD like activity by prion protein itself causes the observed enhancement in resistance.

4.2.1.2 DAF-16/FoxO

Thus DAF-16/FoxO, a transcription factor and one of the common and major oxidative stress mediators in *C. elegans*, serves as an endpoint for *daf-2* [10, 85, 231] and SIR-2.1 [215], as well as for JKK-1/JNK-1, for DAF-7/IGF-β and TOR/DAF-15 signalling pathways, which more or less all respond to different forms of environmental stress [20],. This transcription factor was knocked out to see if the advantage in Paraquat resistance by prion protein expressing strains would be lost. On the contrary, the gap between prion protein expressing and those which do not in Paraquat resistance increased (3.4.2). Hence, an involvement of DAF-16/FoxO could have definitely been excluded.

Discussion

Paradoxically, all *daf-16* lacking strains had a stronger resistance to Paraquat than those which do express the transcription factor. It was Hoogewijs, however, who showed that the deletion of *daf-2* leads to the expected increase in all SOD levels, since *daf-16* becomes disinhibited, but the deletion of *daf-16* also leads to a similar effect, most especially to an increase in *sod-1* and *sod-5* gene expression [86], the ones probably mostly needed in this experimental setup. The reason for this paradoxically elevated SOD gene expression remains obscure. Furthermore, a difference in nematode flight rates was observed with the *daf-16* lacking animals weaker in responding to the stress in terms of moving, and therefore with a lower flight rate of nematodes to the edge of the plate. These cases are usually excluded from analysis because of death by desiccation instead of by the initial stressing factor (2.2.3.2). This resulted in a more extensive sample of evaluated worms.

Another obscure feature observed was a further enhancement of Paraquat resistance in prion protein expressing lines lacking DAF-16/FoxO compared to controls. An explanation is so far missing. It might be correlated that a deletion of such a major stress regulator highlights the stress regulating effects of PrP^C, or it might be caused by a more extensive worm sample because of the weaker flight rate.

4.2.1.3 SKN-1/Nrf-2

Another important mediator in stress resistance in *C. elegans* is a transcription factor named SKN-1/Nrf-2 [94, 97, 145, 156, 205, 233], which induces stress responsive genes and also interacts with DAF-16/FoxO while it is the endpoint of the p38/MAPK signalling pathway [20]. Thus SKN-1/Nrf-2 ribosomal transcription was inhibited by RNAi, but again the gap in Paraquat resistance between prion protein expressing strains and those which do not was preserved or even enlarged (3.4.3), indicating that PrP^C induced advantage in Paraquat resistance is not mediated by SKN-1/Nrf-2. Similar to the DAF-16/FoxO knock-out strain, all lines of the SKN-1/Nrf-2 strain showed an enhanced resistance to Paraquat if compared to those normally expressing the transcription factor. Although there is no published data a similar explanation as the one used to account for the DAF-16/FoxO worm can be assumed, although opposite behavior with SKN-1/Nrf-2 mutants showing increased sensitivity towards Paraquat is described as well [5].

The flight rate of the SKN-1/Nrf-2 strain is lower then in the RNAi untreated versions causing a more extensive worm sample than usual. Similar to DAF-16/FoxO strains, the prion protein effect on Paraquat resistance was further highlighted; again we would suggest the same hypothesis as above (4.2.1.2), since an evidenced explanation has not yet been put forward.

4.2.1.4 SOD knock-out

As the major stress responsive mediators were excluded from this observed PrP^C mediated increase in Paraquat resistance, it was searched whether the resistance was mediated by increased SOD activity, either of the endogenous SODs or due to an intrinsic SOD activity of PrP^C. As Paraquat is an externally affiliated stressor producing $O_2^{\cdot-}$ on direct chemical interactions which cannot cross membranes, therefore producing different $O_2^{\cdot-}$ pools [98], intracellular and extracellular SOD forms were considered sparing mitochondrial SOD forms of *C. elegans*. Besides, SOD-1 makes up for about 80% of the total SOD activity in *C. elegans* [59]. Although opposing data is available regarding this subject, Tawe et al. (1998) identified the intracellular Cu/Zn-SOD, namely SOD-1, and the mitochondrial Mn-SOD, namely SOD-3, to be elevated in Paraquat environment [199], while Yanase et al. (2009) [230] and Oeda et al. (2001) [141] describe SOD-1 as the major player. And indeed *sod-1* seems to be play a responsible role in our experimental model, since all strains almost completely lose their ability to resist and detoxify Paraquat induced $O_2^{\cdot-}$ when *sod-1* is knocked-out and, most importantly, the gap between prion protein expressing and non-expressing lines is closed (3.4.4). In line with a recent report by Doonan et al. (2008) [59], SOD-5, an additional intracellular Cu/Zn-SOD and the extracellular Cu/Zn-SOD SOD-4, seem to be irrelevant for baseline resistance of *C. elegans* against Paraquat. However, these two SODs seem to be of major relevance for the additional positive effect of PrP^C on Paraquat resistance in the nematode, as *sod-4* or *sod-5* deficient lines expressing PrP^C seem to have the same lifespan pattern under Paraquat stress as those which do not express PrP^C but are also *sod-4* or *sod-5* deficient.

Therefore, it can be concluded that *sod-1* is the major responsible SOD for Paraquat resistance and it is also responsible for the enhanced resistance in PrP^C strains. However, based on our data, we propose that PrP^C cannot directly influence SOD-1, but rather uses SOD-4 and SOD-5 to modulate and boost SOD-1 activity. At least for *sod-4*, such a theory has already been recently published by Doonan et al. (2008) [59] and Weinkove et al. (2006) [218], hence SOD-4 is expressed in two different forms by alternative splicing, one which is membrane bound and one which is free in the extracellular space. The membrane bound SOD-4 kind produces H_2O_2, which then crosses the extracellular membrane to activate an insulin/insulin-like growth factor-like signalling (IIS) causing a retention of DAF-16. No such ideas have postulated so far for *sod-5* but, as with *sod-4*, these SODs still very unknown and undefined, with the promise of new and fascinating insights to come.

As already mentioned, the possibility of the generally extracellularly located PrP^C interacting with other enzymes is well established (1.2.4). As for its localisation in lipid rafts and being endocytosed by a clathrin-dependent mechanism, it requires an adaptor protein. Possible interactions of caveolin-1 and downstream responding Fyn- or Src-tyrosine-kinase have been highly investigated [200].

Furthermore, STI1 is also a hotly debated interactor with the endocytosed PrP^C, leading to an activation of ERK1/2 [7, 40]. The possible interaction between *sod-4* and *sod-5* could be similar. For *sod-5* being located intracellularly, one can think of endocytosed prion protein or possible cytosolic isoforms of PrP^C interacting with SOD-5 causing a downstream cascade, leading to a change in SOD-1, which in turn causes increased cellular resistance towards Paraquat. Or for SOD-4, it is one legitimate hypothesis that extracellular located PrP^C activates membrane bound SOD-4, leading to an activation of IIS or possibly other unknown enzymes. If it would cause an activation of IIS, then the additional protection against Paraquat is not caused through the retention of DAF-16 through IIS (as previously written), since our results strongly propose that DAF-16 is of no relevance for PrP^C to cause additional Paraquat protection (4.2.1.2).

4.2.1.5 Prion protein and copper

As one discusses the possible function of PrP^C in oxidative stress management, one cannot ignore the theories of PrP^C interacting with copper (Cu^{2+}). The N-terminal region of prion protein between residues 51 to 91 contain an octapeat region composed of aa-sequence PHGGGWGQ repeated 4 times, offering a binding site for Cu^{2+} [29, 88] while the coordination of four Cu^{2+} is achieved by imidazole and amide-nitrogen substitutes in HGGGW [38, 39, 212], and of another two by His-96 and His-111 [95, 100]. The discussed ,but not definitely proven, effects of binding copper are diverse and hotly debated. For on, it is suggested that PrP^C modulates copper transportation from extra- to intracellular lumen with the help of different affinities by pH fluctuations between the different lumen [115, 134, 146, 147, 226] only illustrated, however, *in vitro*. Other studies [34, 95, 100, 135, 157, 192, 212, 229] showed that Cu^{2+} changes recombinant PrP^C conformation and affects the folding of recombinant prion protein. However, more reliable *in vivo* data is quite rare [159]. Copper also seems to facilitate its self-association *in vitro* [220, 221]. The most interesting part of this context regarding the above discussed function of PrP^C in SOD modulation is its putative role in antioxidant capacity. It has been an often postulated thesis that the presumed role of PrP^C in regulating SOD levels or its activity is connected to the binding of copper at the N-terminal octarepeat region, and is proven *in vitro* [32, 161, 162] and *in vivo* [29, 82, 107, 228] on human and murine PrP^C. Just as well it has been suggested for *in vitro* and *in vivo* models that the binding of copper itself exerts an antioxidant effect by scavenging the putative ROS, namely Cu^{2+} [27, 32, 235].

Alternatively, it was suggested that Cu^{2+} induces endocytosis of PrP^C while triggering stress pathways for antioxidative defence [211], which would explain why a decreased level of glutathione reductase and other antioxidant enzymes has been detected in prion protein lacking mice [161, 223]. Interestingly, oxidative stress and copper exposure also appear to induce PrP^C

Discussion

expression, while heavy metal responding sequences have been identified on the *Prnp* gene [209, 210]. Therefore, it was expected that the deletion of the octarepeat region in our PrP^C - *C. elegans* model has in some way a diminishing effect on Paraquat resistance, but the opposite was observed. The Δ8 strain shows a similar Paraquat resistance as the strains transformed with full-length PrP^C (3.4.5), demonstrating that the loss of the octarepeat region, and, consequently, the loss of four potential copper ion binding sides, is of no effect on prion protein induced Paraquat resistance. However, the deletion of the octarepeat region still leaves other binding sides at His -96 and His-111, which were recently shown in an *in vitro* study to have a higher affinity to Cu^{2+} than the octarepeat region, likely being of greater value [109]. However, data like this is achieved *in vitro*; in our *C. elegans* model we abdicated to delete or change the aa-sequence at His-96 and His-111, as this part is known to be crucial for PrP^C and changes leading to toxic versions[178]. On the other hand, it also has to be mentioned that there is contradicting data regarding this subject. For example, a strong piece of evidence for a role of PrP^C in Cu^{2+} metabolism would be a correlation between PrP^C expression levels and the cellular copper content. However, there is published data suggesting that the cellular copper content drops to 10% of normal in *Prn-p$^{0/0}$* mice [29], or, in a subsequent study from the same authors, to 50% of normal compared to wildtype animals [82]. Furthermore, other scientist were unable to see any differences in copper content in brain tissue from wildtype, *Prn-p$^{0/0}$* mice as well as in Tga20 mice which overexpress PrP^C by 10-fold using mass spectrometry [216].

A different approach was tried by culturing *C. elegans* in a non-toxic $CuSO_4$ enriched environment. This was done in an attempt to enhance the effect on Paraquat resistance seen by prion protein expressing lines. The results, however, were not exploitable, showing a totally incoherent pattern (3.7) for which no explanation could, as of yet, be found. However, another fact to consider when discussing possible interactions of PrP^C with copper metabolism, is the model *C. elegans* itself. If we assume that PrP^C induces the expression, translation or activation of *sod-1*, it has to be mentioned that SOD-1 needs to be loaded with copper as a redox partner in order to function and, that different species have different ways to do so. The human being is known to have two ways of transporting Cu^{2+}, one CCS dependent and the other CCS independent [98]. For the CCS independent way it is known that it relies on glutathione for activity [42]. However, the copper carrier for this pathway has not yet been identified, nor has an explanation been found for how the essential disulfide bond oxidation is occurring. For the CCS dependent way, a chaperone, the CCS, is needed. The reason for this is that SOD-1 has a low affinity to Cu^{2+}, while free copper is highly cytotoxic, and strong chelators are needed to bind toxic free copper [98]. As mentioned, the human possesses another CCS independent way to load SOD-1 with copper ions. For example, it has been put forward that SOD-1 compensates for its low affinity through a faster protein folding kinetic

Discussion

[163]. *C. elegans*, on the other hand, does not command such a CCS, leaving only a copper independent way. It is discussed that GSH may function as a copper donator, which was shown in a yeast model expressing *C. elegans* SODs, but this activation is only partial as it is expressed in humans as well [98]. However, it is known that worm SODs do not require an oxidation for activation because of a different amino acid sequence which destabilizes the disulfide bond and enables them to oxidize spontaneously [98]. It is, therefore, not clear if *C. elegans* is able to express the same relationship between PrP^C, SOD-1 and Cu^{2+} as observed in mammalian organisms, and further research has to be done.

4.2.1.6 SOD enzyme assay

To further analyze the involvement of PrP^C in SOD-1 activity levels, a different test approach was used, a SOD Enzyme Assay (3.9). Observing the results under no Paraquat influence, it is seen that the activities of cyanide inhibited and ethanol inhibited added together do not sum up to the total activity seen in the untreated version. Regarding this event, the supplying company BIOMOL GmbH was questioned, which informed us that this phenomenon is probably due to a complex interaction and inter-inhibition of the respective SODs. Therefore, a direct comparison between the lines and activities is not possible, except on a relative basis. The lower overall activity of SODs in the worms tested under Paraquat conditions might be due to the fact that the nematode reduces its enzyme translation ability in the endphase of its being [199]. What, however, becomes obvious is that the prion protein expressing lines rely in large part on Cu/Zn-SOD, especially under Paraquat stress, where PrP line 2 shows a clear shift towards Cu/Zn-SODs, while PrP line 1 has this extreme relation from the beginning. Likewise, plasmid line also shows a shift, except it is towards Mn-SODs instead of towards Cu/Zn-SODs under stress conditions. While the *sod-1* deficient line clearly indicates that SOD-1 is the major player under Paraquat conditions, with almost no SOD activity at all and which in turn cannot be compensated by SOD-4 or SOD-5. While the overall activity under no stress conditions in SOD-1 knock-out line is comparable to plasmid line. The reason for the initial differences between the strains expressing prion protein is probably due to differences in the initial stress level of the worm populations. As PrP line 1 already shows this extreme shift towards Cu/Zn-SODs still missing Paraquat, it is most likely that the populations were contaminated through the culturing process, causing oxidative stress a long time before Paraquat was added.

Thus we conclude that PrP^C probably leads to an enhanced activity of SOD-1, while the missing compensation of SOD-4/-5 in SOD-1 knock-out line most likely indicates that SOD-4/-5 rather serves as a regulator of SOD-1 than as a direct enhancer of Paraquat resistance by its own detoxifying mechanisms.

Discussion

4.2.1.7 Intermediate summary

Summing it up at this point, we were able to show that the expression of huPrP^C in the nematode *C. elegans* has a protective effect against oxidative stress in terms of $O_2^{\cdot-}$, while this effect in our model system is not related to the octapeptide repeat region of PrP^C. Furthermore the observed effects do not require two of the major stress signalling pathways of *C. elegans*, DAF-16/FoxO and SKN-1/Nrf-2. However, the major player in Paraquat resistance was proven to be SOD-1, while SOD-4 and SOD-5 are not involved in the basic anti-stress mechanism, but are most likely responsible for the additional resistance of PrP^C expressing lines compared to non-expressing, suggesting that the benefits induced by PrP^C under Paraquat stress are probably mediated by SOD-4 and/or SOD-5 by inducing or activating SOD-1.

4.2.2 Other stressors

4.2.2.1 Hydrogen peroxide

A common mistake in testing the function of PrP^C in a model organism or cell culture is to take results from specific radical species and generalize them to all kinds of oxidative stress models. There are several specific kinds of ROS which all need a specific cellular answer to be dealt with. It is actually incorrect to talk about ROS in matters of oxidative stress, since it is no requirement for a radical to be oxygen derived, making RS a more accurate term. Scilicet, a radical, is defined by either acting as an e$^-$ donor or acceptor, which either forms covalent bridges with other radicals or, if that is not possible, new radicals result in a manner of chain reaction. The same happens when $O_2^{\cdot-}$ caused by Paraquat are detoxified by SODs. What results is not an elimination of the radical but simply a turn over in another less reactive agent. In this case, $O_2^{\cdot-}$ is turned into H_2O_2, which needs further detoxification by glutathione, where GSH becomes oxidized to GSSG, or by catalase, an enzyme which is very rarely expressed in neurons and probably functions most likely by a two step mechanism using $Fe^{3+/2+}$, or by recently detected peroxiredoxins, which are homodimers and contain no prosthetic group but depend on cysteine as their active site (all reviewed in [80]).

Thus it was tested whether the expression of PrP^C not only manipulates the resistance against superoxide anions (4.2.1), but also against hydrogen peroxide, since it was described that a lack of PrP^C in neurons of PrP$^{0/0}$ mice have a decreased level of glutathione reductase and an increased susceptibility to H_2O_2 [223]. However, in our models, a different tendency, but one of no statistical significance, was observed, with one of the prion protein expressing lines having a lower resistance than controls (3.8). In figure 33 a similar pattern is observed with *sod-1* deficient line having a significantly decreased lifespan compared to controls, but also with one of the PrP^C expressing lines

Discussion

being significantly reduced in lifespan. Overall, both figures, and therefore both approaches, show that the expression of PrP^C decreases the resistance against H_2O_2 slightly. This might be explainable by the following hypothesis: if the additional expression of PrP^C in *C. elegans* really enhances activity or expression/translation pattern of *sod-1*, then do those strains also have a higher advent of H_2O_2 compared to controls, which then more quickly overstresses the detoxifying mechanisms, especially if the worm is pushed by H_2O_2. On the other hand, both approaches show the *sod-1* lacking strain as having a lower resistance compared to controls which do not express PrP^C. This suggests that the lack of an additional production of H_2O_2 by deletion of *sod-1* does not help the organism. However, it also has to be seen that H_2O_2 is not completely disarmed, but causes other oxidative products and other radicals, like superoxide anions. For the *sod-1* deficient line, however, it is almost impossible to handle this stressor as seen in our Paraquat results (3.4.4). Regarding this partially inconsistent data, it can, as a matter of course, also be assumed that the trials protocol is neither sensitive nor specific enough to work out possible differences. Indeed, it was a laborious path to come up with a protocol which was able to show any usable results at all since *C. elegans* is highly sensitive to the smallest changes in H_2O_2 concentrations, which is also the reason why two approaches are presented here. The significant and very obvious decrease in hydrogen peroxide resistance of all DAF-16/FoxO deleted lines compared to controls (figure 32), which is in unison with published data [218], shows the correctness of the protocol.

4.2.2.2 Heavy metal ions

Besides the above mentioned toxins, it is also the heavy metal ions themselves which are used by most ROS detoxifying enzymes, and, in high concentrations, causes oxidative stress [80]. Heavy metal ions, like Cu^{2+} or $Fe^{3+/2+}$, are radicals which need to be bound by enzymes where they act as their active site or are scavenged to not cause any harm. However, if the organism's threshold is reached, this can result in the generation of toxic reactive oxygen species like the hydroxyl radical (•OH) [228]. The accumulation of Cu^{2+} and the thereby resulting oxidative stress has also already been associated with several neurodegenerative disease like Alzheimer's Disease (AD), where the responsible Amyloid Precursor Protein (APP) contains a copper binding domain [43, 224]. In *C. elegans*, heavy metal caused oxidative stress is primarily handled by JNK-1, which is activated by JKK-1, MKK7 and MEK-1, and also uses the downstream DAF-16/FoxO for responsive gene transcription, including SODs, catalase and GSH [214]. However, as we tested the influence of Cu^{2+} on PrP^C expressing lines and controls, no difference in resistance was measured. Although in figure 30 there are statistical differences between the lines, the additional dotted grey line clearly illustrates that this is only caused by the final diffuse variable spread of the four strains beyond 156 hours, which includes less then 20% of the overall population. If data is calculated only for 156 hours, it shows no statistically significant difference. Although we did not explicitly test for the JNK-1 pathway it can be assumed that PrP^C does not interact with the JNK-1 pathway and *C. elegans*' tolerance against heavy metal ions.

4.2.2.3 Heat stress

Another common approach to investigate the behaviour of *C. elegans* under minatory conditions is to expose them to thermal heat. Heat tolerance is mainly mediated by the heat shock factor family (HSF), which acts as transcriptional regulator for several heat shock proteins (Hsp) [120]. These Hsps enhance survival by binding to misfolded or denatured proteins and targeting these for refolding or for degradation. However, if a certain limit is exceeded, programmed cell death, apoptosis, is induced [149]. HSFs, mainly HSF-1 out of a family comprising four isoforms, also is involved in the development [19] and longevity of *C. elegans* [50, 143], or in regulation of its immunity towards bacteria [181, 182]. It is controlled and activated by the common stress pathways *daf-2* [181, 182], SIR-2.1 in interaction with 14-3-3 proteins [215] or by JNK-1 [143] which all have in common that they act over DAF-16/FoxO. In our experimental setting we were unable to show a difference in behavior between prion protein and non-prion protein lines (3.5). Although there has been a statistical difference between plasmid line and PrP line 1 (figure 26), or between Δ8 and PrP line 2 and plasmid line (figure 29), this still falls in the inaccuracy of the protocol, which allows us to conclude that PrP^C, even if fully translated or with an N-terminal deletion, has no influence on heat tolerance in *C. elegans,* while we were able to confirm that DAF-16/FoxO is of great importance in dealing with elevated temperatures (figure 27). If we look back and remember our argument that PrP^C most likely interacts with *sod-1* activity in the nematode, while prion protein shows no additional effect in heat stress, the deletion of *sod-1* should be of no importance in this setting, which has been confirmed in figure 28 as well. Taken together, these results argue against an interaction of PrP^C with common stress signalling pathways analyzed here.

4.2.3 Dye fill

As we were able to observe an increased resistance of prion protein expressing strains against the chemical toxin Paraquat, but not against other stressors. We were to ensure that this advantage is not due to defects in uptake of the toxin through the chemosensory apparatus of *C. elegans*. *C. elegans* has 302 neurons of which 60 contain sensory cilia. However, only 12 neurons form the so called amphids, a pair of lateral sensilla in the head and tail which are the principal sensory organs [6]. If those sensory organs are impaired, for example, through a defect in cilia movement, the major result is an increased resistance against chemotoxins, while resistance towards other stressor like heat remain unchanged [68, 69]. A dye fill test is an effective way to illustrate the function of

Discussion

the amphids, which, in our case, were proven to be successfully functioning in all strains (3.10). Therefore, increased Paraquat resistance is not due to an impaired uptake of the toxin.

4.3 PrP^C and its role in natural lifespan

One can assume that stress resistance and longevity are based on common mechanisms and factors, or that the adaption of metabolic processes to environmental changes markedly influences lifespan [20]. While the major signalling pathway for stress and longevity control is the *daf-2* or IIS pathway [167] or by *age-1*, which is always mentioned separately but does not stand for a separate signalling pathway, but for a kinase subunit of DAF-2 [14]. Besides its downstream control of DAF-16/FoxO through phosphorylation and repression of the mentioned by DAF-2, it is also a complicated interaction described with other stress, and therefore longevity, regulators [205], where it has been reported that SKN-1/Nrf-2 not only functions as a lifespan and stress mediator but, in parallel, is partly controlled by DAF-2. The case is similar for HSF-1, which was already mentioned in regards to tolerance against elevated temperatures (4.2.2) and is well proven to extend or shorten *C. elegans* lifespan depending on over- or underexpression [137]. SIR-2.1, on the other hand, is already described above as being partly controlled by DAF-2, and has been proven to act independently in terms of lifespan modulation, where it mainly controls the expression of *abu-11*, a member of prion protein-like glutamine/asparagines rich proteins which aid protein folding in the ER [215]. A direct link between endogenous production of ROS has been made by mutations in mitochondrial enzymes, e.g. isp-1 (iron sulphur protein), a part of mitochondrial complex III resulting in lower oxygen consumption. Lower endogenous production of ROS increases lifespan [62]. Differing from this are findings regarding SODs, e.g. mice expressing a *sod-2*$^{+/-}$ pattern, where being exposed to a higher volume of oxidative stress in terms of O_2^- coming from the mitochondria does not show an decreased lifespan [126, 207], while mice overexpressing *sod-1* and *sod-3* show no increase [91]. These results are also in unison with results obtained from *C. elegans* where, on one hand, increased levels of SOD-1, -2 and -3 were observed in long lived animals, but the inhibition of the same by RNAi showed no impact on the natural lifespan [232]. Also, nematodes with a deletion of *sod-1* showed no impact on lifespan, yet had a marked impact on Paraquat resistance [144]. This is also a result we confirmed in our lifespan experiments, where the deletion of the *sod-1* gene did not influence the nematode's life expectancy (figure 12). However, the deletion of DAF-16/FoxO (figure 13) and the inhibition of translation by RNAi of SKN-1/Nrf-2 (figure 14) showed a severe abatement of lifespan, a result which supports the above mentioned literature.

Discussion

If the prion protein expressing lines were compared with controls (wildtype, plasmid line) a double-edged effect was observed, first with an earlier onset of the age induced dying phase in prion protein lines, but also including a second and milder decline when a population size of about 50% was reached (figures 7-9), enabling the prion protein strains to catch up to its controls, the result being an almost identical maximum lifespan. This effect might be explainable regarding the initial expression, correct trafficking and the implementation of the correct function of an additional protein, namely PrP^C, as it causes aadditional stress to the healthy young worm, while the function of PrP^C at this point in an healthy young nematode causes no further advantages. However, if *C. elegans* is exposed to ageing processes and deterioration, PrP^C might support the worm in keeping up correct cell functions, therefore causing milder population reduction and a catch up to controls. This is nicely illustrated by figure 9, which shows the slopes at each lifespan point, clearly displaying almost the same maximum slopes in all lines, with PrP^C expressing lines having a two day earlier inflection point compared to controls initiating the catch-up race.

This was not to be seen in lifespan statistics of the octapeptides deficient strain, which showed a very similar pattern to controls (figure 13), hence the proposal that the nematode carrying the N-terminal modified (51-91)PrP^C does not exert the same lifespan behavior as nematodes with a non modified PrP^C, suggesting that the effect of PrP^C is lost by this deletion. However, this conflicts with the results discussed in context with Paraquat resistance (4.2.1), where the octapeptides missing strain is able to exhibit the same behavior as unchanged prion protein. These results indeed leave us marvelling, hoping for an explanation which cannot be given at this point, but opens a wide field of further research. It most likely can be assumed that during oxidative stress and lifespan different genes, and also different signalling pathways, are activated. This would explain why, for example, there are contradictory results regarding effects about SODs on lifespan, and would give insight about the importance of the octarepeat region of PrP^C. As already mentioned, the octarepeat region is mostly attributed to interaction with copper ions,. However, the discussed features above (4.2.1) are also strongly abnegated by other authors [222], e.g. Waggoner et al. (2000) who argue that there is no difference in copper content in neurons of WT and PrP^C deficient mice brain homogenates [216]. Similar results were found where, in a yeast model, no difference of copper utilization was found between prion protein expressing and non-expressing [116]. Others also argue against PrP^C being directly [102, 163] or indirectly [92, 216] involved in SOD regulation. While the influence of SOD on lifespan, as discussed above, also remains hotly debated, with many taking a position contrary to our results. Paul et al. (1998), for example, showed an severe influence of SODs on lifespan in Drosophila melanogaster [146]. This problem can be best highlighted by publications regarding SOD mimetcs, Euk-134 and Euk-8, with Sampayo et al. (2003) publishing data showing a lifespan extension in *C. elegans* [173, 174] and Keaney et al. (2004) showing the opposite [105] all within a seven months time frame. What I intend with this argument is not to prove or disprove one of these authors, but to show the problems and often contrary results that often appear, even only slightly differing experimental settings, from which I conclude that we are facing very complex mechanisms which, at this point, are difficult to fully explicate. They do, however, provide questions that beg for further research and investigation,.

4.4 Conclusion and outlook

It was the objective of this work to investigate the physiologic function of PrP^C, specifically the influence of PrP^C in management of oxidative stress (1.4). Now, at the end of this work, the following can be stated:

The expression and inheritance of human PrP^C in *C. elegans* is successfully achieved. PrP^C causes an increased stress resistance against Paraquat, a producer of superoxide radicals, in *C. elegans*. There is no advantage or disadvantage for *C. elegans* in expressing prion protein against other stressors like heat, hydrogen peroxide or copper, nor does it have a major impact on lifespan. In *C. elegans,* $huPrP^C$ does most likely not depend on the octarepeat domain to exert its function, and is therefore presumably independent of copper. It was shown that PrP^C depends on sod-1, sod-2 and sod-5 to exert its function in oxidative stress management. While in this scenario sod-1 is most likely the direct disarmer of superoxide radicals, it is sod-4 and sod-5 which act as regulator of sod-1and which, most importantly, are being controlled by PrP^C.

However, many questions remain, we still cannot provide detail information about possible pathways and direct interactions. I also acknowledge that the interconnection between PrP^C and SOD, such as that illustrated here, may not be the only one for PrP^C. Prevalent literature opens a wide field of interactions and interconnections for PrP^C. Here, only one of many interplays of PrP^C have been described. However, *C. elegans* model systems probably are one of the most convenient systems to further investigate the protein mystery which PrP^C provides to the scientific world. The field is open for various RNAi experiments with inhibition of diverse enzymes, or for oral infection with pathogenous PrP^{Sc}, etc. In addition, further specific methods are of interest. For example RT-PCR, like our cooperative partners at the University of Freiburg, Dr. rer. nat. Bettina Schulze and PD Dr. rer. nat. Ekkehard Schulze have initially done, are of major interest. Also, gene array experiments in which activation of various genes can be shown are of interest and remain to be established.

Discussion

PrP^C therefore remains a mystery to the scientific world. Prion protein is the underlying cause of a wide variety of diseases in humans and animals including zoonosis. Moreover, prion protein was evaluated as a bioterroristic threat in 2002 by the US Department of Agriculture [35]. Therefore, the scientific community has an obligation to understand the patterns of this disease. The investigation of PrP^C is one of many steps which need to be taken but definitely one that cannot overstepped.

5 Summary

The cellular prion protein (PrP^C) is a conserved glycoprotein predominantly expressed in neurons, glial and lymphatic cells. It is associated with the broad group of prion protein diseases in which PrP^C becomes misfolded either by inoculation of infectious Scrapie prion protein (PrP^{Sc}) or by spontaneously mutated or inherited pathological prion protein. This creates an inimitable pathogenesis first described by Griffith, driven forward by Prusiner in 1982, the protein only hypothesis in which neither DNA (deoxyribonucleic acid) nor RNA (ribonucleic acid) are needed to cause disease outbreak unlike virus or bacteria. However, the purpose of PrP^C in living cells is still enigmatic.

To elucidate on its cellular function, especially that of its strongly debated function in oxidative stress resistance, the genetic information of human PrP^C was injected in the nematode *Caenorhabditis elegans* (*C. elegans*) by integrating it on an extrachromosomal plasmid. Inserted PrP^C was controlled by the promoter *sel-12* (Suppressor/Enhancer gene of Lin12) and therefore ubiquitously expressed. It was co-expressed with a green fluorescenting protein (GFP) and the thermoselective worm gene *pha-1* (defective pharynx development) for verification of correct inheritance of the previously injected plasmid.

While Western blot experiments showed correct expression and approved glycolysation of PrP^C, it was for GFP imaging to show an ubiquitary expression pattern. By tagging GFP directly to *Prnp* (gene of PrP^C), prion protein appeared to be correctly localized at membranic structures.

C. elegans strains expressing PrP^C were compared with controls of which one strain was carrying an empty plasmid and wildtype in a diverse variety of lifespan experiments. Under non stressful conditions, nematodes expressing PrP^C had an initially earlier onset of death than controls. However, after population size shrank to about 50%, PrP^C expressing strains were able to catch up again and even overtake controls in average lifespan. This suggests an advantage in handling ageing processes, which are mostly of oxidative damage, while the additional expression of PrP^C obviously acts as a stressor, causing an earlier onset of death. For further investigation, strains were exposed to Paraquat causing the creation of superoxide anions. PrP^C expressing nematodes showed a significant advantage compared to controls. As interaction of PrP^C with *C. elegans* stress pathways were excluded by testing DAF-16/FoxO knock-out and SKN1 RNAi (both oxidative stress regulated transcription factors) inhibited strains in a simulative manner, we suggest that PrP^C

Summary

directly or indirectly influences SOD (superoxide dismutase) detoxification processes. However, expression of PrP^C showed no effect in handling other stressors like hydrogen peroxide, heat and copper ions intoxication.

To further differentiate this phenomenon, different SOD knock-out lines were tested in combination with prion protein expression and non-expression. It became evident that Paraquat resistance is only achieved by expression of SOD-1. However, advantageous resistance of PrP^C expressing strains is only achieved via SOD-4 and SOD-5 expression. It can be inferred that additional resistance of prion protein strains is caused by SOD-1 overexpression regulated by SOD-4 and SOD-5.

A different approach besides lifespan testing was taken through the use of SOD Enzyme Assay, a method used to determine the activity of Cu/Zn-SODs (SOD-1,-4,-5) and Mn-SODs (SOD-2,-3). These results could be interpreted as prion protein expressing lines shift towards Cu/Zn-SODs when exposed to Paraquat while controls do not. Besides by using the *sod-1* knock-out line, it was illustrated that SOD-4/-5 are not able to compensate the loss, therefore implementing a control instead of a detoxifying function. However, further experiments to increase reliability of the assay are necessary.

Since an increased resistance towards Paraquat is not only described by modifying stress pathways but also by changes in chemosensory neurons of *C. elegans*, the unrestricted functionality was proven by dye fill procedure.

Hence, it can be concluded that *C. elegans* was established as a new model system in prion protein research. It was further proven that human cellular PrP^C is capable of improving resistance of *C. elegans* against superoxide anions, while it is shown that PrP^C modifies the expression or activity level of SOD-1 by interaction with SOD-4 and SOD-5, which, in turn, act as regulator enzymes for the first mentioned. This is most likely done by a *C. elegans* atypical stress signalling pathway.

The need for further analysis on the function of PrP^C and the pathogenesis of PrP^{Sc} *C. elegans* opens a wide field of further investigations and different methods. Subjects such as the feeding of infectious prion protein, silencing of genes by RNAi (inhibitory RNA) or classical methods, e.g. Real-Time-PCR (polymerase chain reaction) and Gene Arrays, should broaden our knowledge in near future.

6 Literature

1. Adler, V., B. Zeiler, V. Kryukov, R. Kascsak, R. Rubenstein, and A. Grossman, Small, highly structured RNAs participate in the conversion of human recombinant PrP(Sen) to PrP(Res) in vitro. J Mol Biol. 1: 47-57.(2003)
2. Albertson, D.G. and J.N. Thomson, The pharynx of Caenorhabditis elegans. Philos Trans R Soc Lond B Biol Sci. 938: 299-325.(1976)
3. Alper, T., W.A. Cramp, D.A. Haig, and M.C. Clarke, Does the agent of scrapie replicate without nucleic acid? Nature. 5090: 764-766.(1967)
4. Alper, T., D.A. Haig, and M.C. Clarke, The exceptionally small size of the scrapie agent. Biochem Biophys Res Commun. 3: 278-284.(1966)
5. An, J.H. and T.K. Blackwell, SKN-1 links C. elegans mesendodermal specification to a conserved oxidative stress response. Genes Dev. 15: 1882-1893.(2003)
6. Apfeld, J. and C. Kenyon, Regulation of lifespan by sensory perception in Caenorhabditis elegans. Nature. 6763: 804-809.(1999)
7. Arantes, C., R. Nomizo, M.H. Lopes, G.N. Hajj, F.R. Lima, and V.R. Martins, Prion protein and its ligand stress inducible protein 1 regulate astrocyte development. Glia. 13: 1439-1449.(2009)
8. Artinger, K.B., N. Fedtsova, J.M. Rhee, M. Bronner-Fraser, and E. Turner, Placodal origin of Brn-3-expressing cranial sensory neurons. J Neurobiol. 4: 572-585.(1998)
9. Askanas, V. and W.K. Engel, Inclusion-body myositis: newest concepts of pathogenesis and relation to aging and Alzheimer disease. J Neuropathol Exp Neurol. 1: 1-14.(2001)
10. Atarashi, R., N. Nishida, K. Shigematsu, S. Goto, T. Kondo, S. Sakaguchi, and S. Katamine, Deletion of N-terminal residues 23-88 from prion protein (PrP) abrogates the potential to rescue PrP-deficient mice from PrP-like protein/doppel-induced Neurodegeneration. J Biol Chem. 31: 28944-28949.(2003)
11. Ayyadevara, S., A. Dandapat, S.P. Singh, H. Benes, L. Zimniak, R.J. Reis, and P. Zimniak, Lifespan extension in hypomorphic daf-2 mutants of Caenorhabditis elegans is partially mediated by glutathione transferase CeGSTP2-2. Aging Cell. 6: 299-307.(2005)
12. Ballerini, C., P. Gourdain, V. Bachy, N. Blanchard, E. Levavasseur, S. Gregoire, P. Fontes, P. Aucouturier, C. Hivroz, and C. Carnaud, Functional implication of cellular prion protein in antigen-driven interactions between T cells and dendritic cells. J Immunol. 12: 7254-7262.(2006)

13. Barmada, S., P. Piccardo, K. Yamaguchi, B. Ghetti, and D.A. Harris, GFP-tagged prion protein is correctly localized and functionally active in the brains of transgenic mice. Neurobiol Dis. 3: 527-537.(2004)
14. Barsyte, D., D.A. Lovejoy, and G.J. Lithgow, Longevity and heavy metal resistance in daf-2 and age-1 long-lived mutants of Caenorhabditis elegans. Faseb J. 3: 627-634.(2001)
15. Basler, K., B. Oesch, M. Scott, D. Westaway, M. Walchli, D.F. Groth, M.P. McKinley, S.B. Prusiner, and C. Weissmann, Scrapie and cellular PrP isoforms are encoded by the same chromosomal gene. Cell. 3: 417-428.(1986)
16. Bastian, F.O., Spiroplasma-like inclusions in Creutzfeldt-Jakob disease. Arch Pathol Lab Med. 13: 665-669.(1979)
17. Bastian, F.O., Spiroplasma as a candidate agent for the transmissible spongiform encephalopathies. J Neuropathol Exp Neurol. 10: 833-838.(2005)
18. Bastian, F.O., S. Dash, and R.F. Garry, Linking chronic wasting disease to scrapie by comparison of Spiroplasma mirum ribosomal DNA sequences. Exp Mol Pathol. 1: 49-56.(2004)
19. Bastian, F.O., D.E. Sanders, W.A. Forbes, S.D. Hagius, J.V. Walker, W.G. Henk, F.M. Enright, and P.H. Elzer, Spiroplasma spp. from transmissible spongiform encephalopathy brains or ticks induce spongiform encephalopathy in ruminants. J Med Microbiol. Pt 9: 1235-1242.(2007)
20. Baumeister, R., E. Schaffitzel, and M. Hertweck, Endocrine signaling in Caenorhabditis elegans controls stress response and longevity. J Endocrinol. 2: 191-202.(2006)
21. Bolton, D.C., M.P. McKinley, and S.B. Prusiner, Molecular characteristics of the major scrapie prion protein. Biochemistry. 25: 5898-5906.(1984)
22. Borchelt, D.R., M. Scott, A. Taraboulos, N. Stahl, and S.B. Prusiner, Scrapie and cellular prion proteins differ in their kinetics of synthesis and topology in cultured cells. J Cell Biol. 3: 743-752.(1990)
23. Borges, V.M., H. Falcao, J.H. Leite-Junior, L. Alvim, G.P. Teixeira, M. Russo, A.F. Nobrega, M.F. Lopes, P.M. Rocco, W.F. Davidson, R. Linden, H. Yagita, W.A. Zin, and G.A. DosReis, Fas ligand triggers pulmonary silicosis. J Exp Med. 2: 155-164.(2001)
24. Bounhar, Y., Y. Zhang, C.G. Goodyer, and A. LeBlanc, Prion protein protects human neurons against Bax-mediated apoptosis. J Biol Chem. 42: 39145-39149.(2001)
25. Brenner, S., The genetics of Caenorhabditis elegans. Genetics. 1: 71-94.(1974)
26. Brown, D.R., Prion and prejudice: normal protein and the synapse. Trends Neurosci. 2: 85-90.(2001)

27. Brown, D.R., C. Clive, and S.J. Haswell, Antioxidant activity related to copper binding of native prion protein. J Neurochem. 1: 69-76.(2001)
28. Brown, D.R., R.S. Nicholas, and L. Canevari, Lack of prion protein expression results in a neuronal phenotype sensitive to stress. J Neurosci Res. 2: 211-224.(2002)
29. Brown, D.R., K. Qin, J.W. Herms, A. Madlung, J. Manson, R. Strome, P.E. Fraser, T. Kruck, A. von Bohlen, W. Schulz-Schaeffer, A. Giese, D. Westaway, and H. Kretzschmar, The cellular prion protein binds copper in vivo. Nature. 6661: 684-687.(1997)
30. Brown, D.R., B. Schmidt, M.H. Groschup, and H.A. Kretzschmar, Prion protein expression in muscle cells and toxicity of a prion protein fragment. Eur J Cell Biol. 1: 29-37.(1998)
31. Brown, D.R., B. Schmidt, and H.A. Kretzschmar, Effects of oxidative stress on prion protein expression in PC12 cells. Int J Dev Neurosci. 8: 961-972.(1997)
32. Brown, D.R., B. Schmidt, and H.A. Kretzschmar, Effects of copper on survival of prion protein knockout neurons and glia. J Neurochem. 4: 1686-1693.(1998)
33. Brown, D.R., W.J. Schulz-Schaeffer, B. Schmidt, and H.A. Kretzschmar, Prion protein-deficient cells show altered response to oxidative stress due to decreased SOD-1 activity. Exp Neurol. 1: 104-112.(1997)
34. Brown, D.R., B.S. Wong, F. Hafiz, C. Clive, S.J. Haswell, and I.M. Jones, Normal prion protein has an activity like that of superoxide dismutase. Biochem J: 1-5.(1999)
35. Brown, P. and C.R. Abee, Working with transmissible spongiform encephalopathy agents. Ilar J. 1: 44-52.(2005)
36. Bueler, H., M. Fischer, Y. Lang, H. Bluethmann, H.P. Lipp, S.J. DeArmond, S.B. Prusiner, M. Aguet, and C. Weissmann, Normal development and behaviour of mice lacking the neuronal cell-surface PrP protein. Nature. 6370: 577-582.(1992)
37. Burnette, W.N., "Western blotting": electrophoretic transfer of proteins from sodium dodecyl sulfate--polyacrylamide gels to unmodified nitrocellulose and radiographic detection with antibody and radioiodinated protein A. Anal Biochem. 2: 195-203.(1981)
38. Burns, C.S., E. Aronoff-Spencer, C.M. Dunham, P. Lario, N.I. Avdievich, W.E. Antholine, M.M. Olmstead, A. Vrielink, G.J. Gerfen, J. Peisach, W.G. Scott, and G.L. Millhauser, Molecular features of the copper binding sites in the octarepeat domain of the prion protein. Biochemistry. 12: 3991-4001.(2002)
39. Burns, C.S., E. Aronoff-Spencer, G. Legname, S.B. Prusiner, W.E. Antholine, G.J. Gerfen, J. Peisach, and G.L. Millhauser, Copper coordination in the full-length, recombinant prion protein. Biochemistry. 22: 6794-6803.(2003)
40. Caetano, F.A., M.H. Lopes, G.N. Hajj, C.F. Machado, C. Pinto Arantes, A.C. Magalhaes, P. Vieira Mde, T.A. Americo, A.R. Massensini, S.A. Priola, I. Vorberg, M.V. Gomez, R.

Linden, V.F. Prado, V.R. Martins, and M.A. Prado, Endocytosis of prion protein is required for ERK1/2 signaling induced by stress-inducible protein 1. J Neurosci. 26: 6691-6702.(2008)

41. Cagampang, F.R., S.A. Whatley, A.L. Mitchell, J.F. Powell, I.C. Campbell, and C.W. Coen, Circadian regulation of prion protein messenger RNA in the rat forebrain: a widespread and synchronous rhythm. Neuroscience. 4: 1201-1204.(1999)

42. Carroll, M.C., J.B. Girouard, J.L. Ulloa, J.R. Subramaniam, P.C. Wong, J.S. Valentine, and V.C. Culotta, Mechanisms for activating Cu- and Zn-containing superoxide dismutase in the absence of the CCS Cu chaperone. Proc Natl Acad Sci U S A. 16: 5964-5969.(2004)

43. Cerpa, W.F., M.I. Barria, M.A. Chacon, M. Suazo, M. Gonzalez, C. Opazo, A.I. Bush, and N.C. Inestrosa, The N-terminal copper-binding domain of the amyloid precursor protein protects against Cu2+ neurotoxicity in vivo. Faseb J. 14: 1701-1703.(2004)

44. Chakrabarti, O. and R.S. Hegde, Functional depletion of mahogunin by cytosolically exposed prion protein contributes to neurodegeneration. Cell. 6: 1136-1147.(2009)

45. Chen, S.G., D.B. Teplow, P. Parchi, J.K. Teller, P. Gambetti, and L. Autilio-Gambetti, Truncated forms of the human prion protein in normal brain and in prion diseases. J Biol Chem. 32: 19173-19180.(1995)

46. Chesebro, B., M. Trifilo, R. Race, K. Meade-White, C. Teng, R. LaCasse, L. Raymond, C. Favara, G. Baron, S. Priola, B. Caughey, E. Masliah, and M. Oldstone, Anchorless prion protein results in infectious amyloid disease without clinical scrapie. Science. 5727: 1435-1439.(2005)

47. Chiarini, L.B., A.R. Freitas, S.M. Zanata, R.R. Brentani, V.R. Martins, and R. Linden, Cellular prion protein transduces neuroprotective signals. Embo J. 13: 3317-3326.(2002)

48. Coitinho, A.S., M.O. Dietrich, A. Hoffmann, O.P. Dall'Igna, D.O. Souza, V.R. Martins, R.R. Brentani, I. Izquierdo, and D.R. Lara, Decreased hyperlocomotion induced by MK-801, but not amphetamine and caffeine in mice lacking cellular prion protein (PrP(C)). Brain Res Mol Brain Res. 2: 190-194.(2002)

49. Cordeiro, Y., F. Machado, L. Juliano, M.A. Juliano, R.R. Brentani, D. Foguel, and J.L. Silva, DNA converts cellular prion protein into the beta-sheet conformation and inhibits prion peptide aggregation. J Biol Chem. 52: 49400-49409.(2001)

50. Cypser, J.R., P. Tedesco, and T.E. Johnson, Hormesis and aging in Caenorhabditis elegans. Exp Gerontol. 10: 935-939.(2006)

51. de Almeida, C.J., L.B. Chiarini, J.P. da Silva, E.S. PM, M.A. Martins, and R. Linden, The cellular prion protein modulates phagocytosis and inflammatory response. J Leukoc Biol. 2: 238-246.(2005)

52. Deleault, N.R., R.W. Lucassen, and S. Supattapone, RNA molecules stimulate prion protein conversion. Nature. 6959: 717-720.(2003)
53. Diarra-Mehrpour, M., S. Arrabal, A. Jalil, X. Pinson, C. Gaudin, G. Pietu, A. Pitaval, H. Ripoche, M. Eloit, D. Dormont, and S. Chouaib, Prion protein prevents human breast carcinoma cell line from tumor necrosis factor alpha-induced cell death. Cancer Res. 2: 719-727.(2004)
54. Dillin, A., D.K. Crawford, and C. Kenyon, Timing requirements for insulin/IGF-1 signaling in C. elegans. Science. 5594: 830-834.(2002)
55. Diringer, H., Sustained viremia in experimental hamster scrapie. Brief report. Arch Virol. 1-2: 105-109.(1984)
56. Diringer, H., Durchbrechen von Speziesbarrieren mit unkonventionellen Viren. Bundesgesundhbl. 10: 435-440.(1990)
57. Diringer, H., Proposed link between transmissible spongiform encephalopathies of man and animals. Lancet. 8984: 1208-1210.(1995)
58. Diringer, H., M. Beekes, M. Ozel, D. Simon, I. Queck, F. Cardone, M. Pocchiari, and J.W. Ironside, Highly infectious purified preparations of disease-specific amyloid of transmissible spongiform encephalopathies are not devoid of nucleic acids of viral size. Intervirology. 4: 238-246.(1997)
59. Doonan, R., J.J. McElwee, F. Matthijssens, G.A. Walker, K. Houthoofd, P. Back, A. Matscheski, J.R. Vanfleteren, and D. Gems, Against the oxidative damage theory of aging: superoxide dismutases protect against oxidative stress but have little or no effect on life span in Caenorhabditis elegans. Genes Dev. 23: 3236-3241.(2008)
60. Drisaldi, B., J. Coomaraswamy, P. Mastrangelo, B. Strome, J. Yang, J.C. Watts, M.A. Chishti, M. Marvi, O. Windl, R. Ahrens, F. Major, M.S. Sy, H. Kretzschmar, P.E. Fraser, H.T. Mount, and D. Westaway, Genetic mapping of activity determinants within cellular prion proteins: N-terminal modules in PrPC offset pro-apoptotic activity of the Doppel helix B/B' region. J Biol Chem. 53: 55443-55454.(2004)
61. Drisaldi, B., R.S. Stewart, C. Adles, L.R. Stewart, E. Quaglio, E. Biasini, L. Fioriti, R. Chiesa, and D.A. Harris, Mutant PrP is delayed in its exit from the endoplasmic reticulum, but neither wild-type nor mutant PrP undergoes retrotranslocation prior to proteasomal degradation. J Biol Chem. 24: 21732-21743.(2003)
62. Feng, J., F. Bussiere, and S. Hekimi, Mitochondrial electron transport is a key determinant of life span in Caenorhabditis elegans. Dev Cell. 5: 633-644.(2001)

63. Finner, H. and M. Roters, Asymptotic comparison of the critical values of step-down and step-up multiple comparison procedures Journal of Statistical Planning and Inference. 1: 11-30.(1998)
64. Fischer, M., T. Rulicke, A. Raeber, A. Sailer, M. Moser, B. Oesch, S. Brandner, A. Aguzzi, and C. Weissmann, Prion protein (PrP) with amino-proximal deletions restoring susceptibility of PrP knockout mice to scrapie. Embo J. 6: 1255-1264.(1996)
65. Ford, M.J., L.J. Burton, H. Li, C.H. Graham, Y. Frobert, J. Grassi, S.M. Hall, and R.J. Morris, A marked disparity between the expression of prion protein and its message by neurones of the CNS. Neuroscience. 3: 533-551.(2002)
66. Ford, M.J., L.J. Burton, R.J. Morris, and S.M. Hall, Selective expression of prion protein in peripheral tissues of the adult mouse. Neuroscience. 1: 177-192.(2002)
67. Forloni, G., S. Iussich, T. Awan, L. Colombo, N. Angeretti, L. Girola, I. Bertani, G. Poli, M. Caramelli, M. Grazia Bruzzone, L. Farina, L. Limido, G. Rossi, G. Giaccone, J.W. Ironside, O. Bugiani, M. Salmona, and F. Tagliavini, Tetracyclines affect prion infectivity. Proc Natl Acad Sci U S A. 16: 10849-10854.(2002)
68. Fujii, M., Y. Matsumoto, N. Tanaka, K. Miki, T. Suzuki, N. Ishii, and D. Ayusawa, Mutations in chemosensory cilia cause resistance to paraquat in nematode Caenorhabditis elegans. J Biol Chem. 19: 20277-20282.(2004)
69. Fujii, M., N. Tanaka, K. Miki, M.N. Hossain, M. Endoh, and D. Ayusawa, Uncoupling of longevity and paraquat resistance in mutants of the nematode Caenorhabditis elegans. Biosci Biotechnol Biochem. 10: 2015-2018.(2005)
70. Gaggelli, E., E. Jankowska, H. Kozlowski, A. Marcinkowska, C. Migliorini, P. Stanczak, D. Valensin, and G. Valensin, Structural characterization of the intra- and inter-repeat copper binding modes within the N-terminal region of "prion related protein" (PrP-rel-2) of zebrafish. J Phys Chem B. 47: 15140-15150.(2008)
71. Gajdusek, D.C., C.J. Gibbs, and M. Alpers, Experimental transmission of a Kuru-like syndrome to chimpanzees. Nature. 5025: 794-796.(1966)
72. Gerstmann, J., Fingeragnosie. Eine umschriebene Störung der Orientierung am eigenen Körper. Wiener klinische Wochenschrift: 1010-1012.(1924)
73. Gerstmann, J., E. Sträussler, and I. Scheinker, Über eine eigenartige hereditär-familiäre Erkrankung des Zentralnervensystems. Zugleich ein Beitrag zur Frage des vorzeitigen lokalen Alterns. ZEITSCHRIFT FUR DIE GESAMTE NEUROLOGIE UND PSYCHIATRIE: 736-762.(1936)
74. Glatzel, M. and A. Aguzzi, PrP(C) expression in the peripheral nervous system is a determinant of prion neuroinvasion. J Gen Virol. Pt 11: 2813-2821.(2000)

75. Granato, M., H. Schnabel, and R. Schnabel, pha-1, a selectable marker for gene transfer in C. elegans. Nucleic Acids Res. 9: 1762-1763.(1994)
76. Gray, A., R.J. Francis, and C.L. Scholtz, Spiroplasma and Creutzfeldt-Jakob disease. Lancet. 8186: 152.(1980)
77. Griffith, J.S., Self-replication and scrapie. Nature. 5105: 1043-1044.(1967)
78. Hadlow, W.J., Scrapie and kuru. Lancet: 289-290.(1959)
79. Halliwell, B., Oxidative stress and neurodegeneration: where are we now? J Neurochem. 6: 1634-1658.(2006)
80. Halliwell, B., Biochemistry of oxidative stress. Biochem Soc Trans. Pt 5: 1147-1150.(2007)
81. Haraguchi, T., S. Fisher, S. Olofsson, T. Endo, D. Groth, A. Tarentino, D.R. Borchelt, D. Teplow, L. Hood, A. Burlingame, and et al., Asparagine-linked glycosylation of the scrapie and cellular prion proteins. Arch Biochem Biophys. 1: 1-13.(1989)
82. Herms, J., T. Tings, S. Gall, A. Madlung, A. Giese, H. Siebert, P. Schurmann, O. Windl, N. Brose, and H. Kretzschmar, Evidence of presynaptic location and function of the prion protein. J Neurosci. 20: 8866-8875.(1999)
83. Herms, J.W., T. Tings, S. Dunker, and H.A. Kretzschmar, Prion protein affects Ca2+-activated K+ currents in cerebellar purkinje cells. Neurobiol Dis. 2: 324-330.(2001)
84. Hertweck, M., C. Gobel, and R. Baumeister, C. elegans SGK-1 is the critical component in the Akt/PKB kinase complex to control stress response and life span. Dev Cell. 4: 577-588.(2004)
85. Honda, Y. and S. Honda, The daf-2 gene network for longevity regulates oxidative stress resistance and Mn-superoxide dismutase gene expression in Caenorhabditis elegans. Faseb J. 11: 1385-1393.(1999)
86. Hoogewijs, D., K. Houthoofd, F. Matthijssens, J. Vandesompele, and J.R. Vanfleteren, Selection and validation of a set of reliable reference genes for quantitative sod gene expression analysis in C. elegans. BMC Mol Biol. 1: 9.(2008)
87. Hope, I.A., Background on Caenorhabditis elegans. C. elegans - A Practical Approach, ed. I.A. Hope. Oxford: Oxford University Press. 1-15.(2005)
88. Hornshaw, M.P., J.R. McDermott, and J.M. Candy, Copper binding to the N-terminal tandem repeat regions of mammalian and avian prion protein. Biochem Biophys Res Commun. 2: 621-629.(1995)
89. Hosono, R., S. Nishimoto, and S. Kuno, Alterations of life span in the nematode Caenorhabditis elegans under monoxenic culture conditions. Exp Gerontol. 3: 251-264.(1989)
90. http://www.wormatlas.org. INTRODUCTION TO C. elegans ANATOMY. [cited.

91. Huang, T.T., E.J. Carlson, A.M. Gillespie, Y. Shi, and C.J. Epstein, Ubiquitous overexpression of CuZn superoxide dismutase does not extend life span in mice. J Gerontol A Biol Sci Med Sci. 1: B5-9.(2000)
92. Hutter, G., F.L. Heppner, and A. Aguzzi, No superoxide dismutase activity of cellular prion protein in vivo. Biol Chem. 9: 1279-1285.(2003)
93. Ikeda, K., N. Kawada, Y.Q. Wang, H. Kadoya, K. Nakatani, M. Sato, and K. Kaneda, Expression of cellular prion protein in activated hepatic stellate cells. Am J Pathol. 6: 1695-1700.(1998)
94. Inoue, H., N. Hisamoto, J.H. An, R.P. Oliveira, E. Nishida, T.K. Blackwell, and K. Matsumoto, The C. elegans p38 MAPK pathway regulates nuclear localization of the transcription factor SKN-1 in oxidative stress response. Genes Dev. 19: 2278-2283.(2005)
95. Jackson, G.S., I. Murray, L.L. Hosszu, N. Gibbs, J.P. Waltho, A.R. Clarke, and J. Collinge, Location and properties of metal-binding sites on the human prion protein. Proc Natl Acad Sci U S A. 15: 8531-8535.(2001)
96. Jansen, W.T., M. Bolm, R. Balling, G.S. Chhatwal, and R. Schnabel, Hydrogen peroxide-mediated killing of Caenorhabditis elegans by Streptococcus pyogenes. Infect Immun. 9: 5202-5207.(2002)
97. Jasper, H., SKNy worms and long life. Cell. 6: 915-916.(2008)
98. Jensen, L.T. and V.C. Culotta, Activation of CuZn superoxide dismutases from Caenorhabditis elegans does not require the copper chaperone CCS. J Biol Chem. 50: 41373-41379.(2005)
99. Johnson, C.J., J.A. Pedersen, R.J. Chappell, D. McKenzie, and J.M. Aiken, Oral transmissibility of prion disease is enhanced by binding to soil particles. PLoS Pathog. 7: e93.(2007)
100. Jones, C.E., S.R. Abdelraheim, D.R. Brown, and J.H. Viles, Preferential Cu2+ coordination by His96 and His111 induces beta-sheet formation in the unstructured amyloidogenic region of the prion protein. J Biol Chem. 31: 32018-32027.(2004)
101. Jones, C.E., M. Klewpatinond, S.R. Abdelraheim, D.R. Brown, and J.H. Viles, Probing copper2+ binding to the prion protein using diamagnetic nickel2+ and 1H NMR: the unstructured N terminus facilitates the coordination of six copper2+ ions at physiological concentrations. J Mol Biol. 5: 1393-1407.(2005)
102. Jones, S., M. Batchelor, D. Bhelt, A.R. Clarke, J. Collinge, and G.S. Jackson, Recombinant prion protein does not possess SOD-1 activity. Biochem J. Pt 2: 309-312.(2005)
103. Kahana, E., M. Alter, J. Braham, and D. Sofer, Creutzfeldt-jakob disease: focus among Libyan Jews in Israel. Science. 120: 90-91.(1974)

104. Kanaani, J., S.B. Prusiner, J. Diacovo, S. Baekkeskov, and G. Legname, Recombinant prion protein induces rapid polarization and development of synapses in embryonic rat hippocampal neurons in vitro. J Neurochem. 5: 1373-1386.(2005)

105. Keaney, M., F. Matthijssens, M. Sharpe, J. Vanfleteren, and D. Gems, Superoxide dismutase mimetics elevate superoxide dismutase activity in vivo but do not retard aging in the nematode Caenorhabditis elegans. Free Radic Biol Med. 2: 239-250.(2004)

106. Kimble, J. and D. Hirsh, The postembryonic cell lineages of the hermaphrodite and male gonads in Caenorhabditis elegans. Dev Biol. 2: 396-417.(1979)

107. Klamt, F., F. Dal-Pizzol, M.J. Conte da Frota, R. Walz, M.E. Andrades, E.G. da Silva, R.R. Brentani, I. Izquierdo, and J.C. Fonseca Moreira, Imbalance of antioxidant defense in mice lacking cellular prion protein. Free Radic Biol Med. 10: 1137-1144.(2001)

108. Klatzo, I., D.C. Gajdusek, and V. Zigas, Pathology of Kuru. Lab Invest. 4: 799-847.(1959)

109. Klewpatinond, M., P. Davies, S. Bowen, D.R. Brown, and J.H. Viles, Deconvoluting the Cu^{2+} binding modes of full-length prion protein. J Biol Chem. 4: 1870-1881.(2008)

110. Kramer, M.L., H.D. Kratzin, B. Schmidt, A. Romer, O. Windl, S. Liemann, S. Hornemann, and H. Kretzschmar, Prion protein binds copper within the physiological concentration range. J Biol Chem. 20: 16711-16719.(2001)

111. La Mendola, D., R.P. Bonomo, S. Caminati, G. Di Natale, S.S. Emmi, O. Hansson, G. Maccarrone, G. Pappalardo, A. Pietropaolo, and E. Rizzarelli, Copper(II) complexes with an avian prion N-terminal region and their potential SOD-like activity. J Inorg Biochem. 2: 195-204.(2009)

112. Laemmli, U.K., Cleavage of structural proteins during the assembly of the head of bacteriophage T4. Nature. 5259: 680-685.(1970)

113. Lau, A.L., A.Y. Yam, M.M. Michelitsch, X. Wang, C. Gao, R.J. Goodson, R. Shimizu, G. Timoteo, J. Hall, A. Medina-Selby, D. Coit, C. McCoin, B. Phelps, P. Wu, C. Hu, D. Chien, and D. Peretz, Characterization of prion protein (PrP)-derived peptides that discriminate full-length PrPSc from PrPC. Proc Natl Acad Sci U S A. 28: 11551-11556.(2007)

114. Leclerc, E., H. Serban, S.B. Prusiner, D.R. Burton, and R.A. Williamson, Copper induces conformational changes in the N-terminal part of cell-surface PrPC. Arch Virol. 11: 2103-2109.(2006)

115. Lee, K.S., A.C. Magalhaes, S.M. Zanata, R.R. Brentani, V.R. Martins, and M.A. Prado, Internalization of mammalian fluorescent cellular prion protein and N-terminal deletion mutants in living cells. J Neurochem. 1: 79-87.(2001)

116. Li, A., J. Dong, and D.A. Harris, Cell surface expression of the prion protein in yeast does not alter copper utilization phenotypes. J Biol Chem. 28: 29469-29477.(2004)

117. Li, A. and D.A. Harris, Mammalian prion protein suppresses Bax-induced cell death in yeast. J Biol Chem. 17: 17430-17434.(2005)
118. Lima, F.R., C.P. Arantes, A.G. Muras, R. Nomizo, R.R. Brentani, and V.R. Martins, Cellular prion protein expression in astrocytes modulates neuronal survival and differentiation. J Neurochem. 6: 2164-2176.(2007)
119. Linden, R., V.R. Martins, M.A. Prado, M. Cammarota, I. Izquierdo, and R.R. Brentani, Physiology of the prion protein. Physiol Rev. 2: 673-728.(2008)
120. Lindquist, S., The heat-shock response. Annu Rev Biochem: 1151-1191.(1986)
121. Lopes, M.H., G.N. Hajj, A.G. Muras, G.L. Mancini, R.M. Castro, K.C. Ribeiro, R.R. Brentani, R. Linden, and V.R. Martins, Interaction of cellular prion and stress-inducible protein 1 promotes neuritogenesis and neuroprotection by distinct signaling pathways. J Neurosci. 49: 11330-11339.(2005)
122. Ma, J., R. Wollmann, and S. Lindquist, Neurotoxicity and neurodegeneration when PrP accumulates in the cytosol. Science. 5599: 1781-1785.(2002)
123. Mallucci, G.R., S. Ratte, E.A. Asante, J. Linehan, I. Gowland, J.G. Jefferys, and J. Collinge, Post-natal knockout of prion protein alters hippocampal CA1 properties, but does not result in neurodegeneration. Embo J. 3: 202-210.(2002)
124. Manson, J., J.D. West, V. Thomson, P. McBride, M.H. Kaufman, and J. Hope, The prion protein gene: a role in mouse embryogenesis? Development. 1: 117-122.(1992)
125. Manson, J.C., A.R. Clarke, M.L. Hooper, L. Aitchison, I. McConnell, and J. Hope, 129/Ola mice carrying a null mutation in PrP that abolishes mRNA production are developmentally normal. Mol Neurobiol. 2-3: 121-127.(1994)
126. Mansouri, A., F.L. Muller, Y. Liu, R. Ng, J. Faulkner, M. Hamilton, A. Richardson, T.T. Huang, C.J. Epstein, and H. Van Remmen, Alterations in mitochondrial function, hydrogen peroxide release and oxidative damage in mouse hind-limb skeletal muscle during aging. Mech Ageing Dev. 3: 298-306.(2006)
127. Masters, C.L. and E.P. Richardson, Jr., Subacute spongiform encephalopathy (Creutzfeldt-Jakob disease). The nature and progression of spongiform change. Brain. 2: 333-344.(1978)
128. Mattei, V., T. Garofalo, R. Misasi, A. Circella, V. Manganelli, G. Lucania, A. Pavan, and M. Sorice, Prion protein is a component of the multimolecular signaling complex involved in T cell activation. FEBS Lett. 1-3: 14-18.(2004)
129. McLennan, N.F., P.M. Brennan, A. McNeill, I. Davies, A. Fotheringham, K.A. Rennison, D. Ritchie, F. Brannan, M.W. Head, J.W. Ironside, A. Williams, and J.E. Bell, Prion protein accumulation and neuroprotection in hypoxic brain damage. Am J Pathol. 1: 227-235.(2004)

130. McNeill, A., Comment on "The codon 129 polymorphism of the prion protein gene influences earlier cognitive performance in Down syndrome subjects"--by Del Bo et al. in J Neurol (2003) 250:688-692. J Neurol. 7: 892-893.(2004)

131. Meggendorfer, F., Clinical and genealogical observations in a case of Jacobs spastic pseudosclerosis. ZEITSCHRIFT FUR DIE GESAMTE NEUROLOGIE UND PSYCHIATRIE: 337-341.(1930)

132. Meyer, R.K., A. Lustig, B. Oesch, R. Fatzer, A. Zurbriggen, and M. Vandevelde, A monomer-dimer equilibrium of a cellular prion protein (PrPC) not observed with recombinant PrP. J Biol Chem. 48: 38081-38087.(2000)

133. Meyer, R.K., M.P. McKinley, K.A. Bowman, M.B. Braunfeld, R.A. Barry, and S.B. Prusiner, Separation and properties of cellular and scrapie prion proteins. Proc Natl Acad Sci U S A. 8: 2310-2314.(1986)

134. Miura, T., A. Hori-i, H. Mototani, and H. Takeuchi, Raman spectroscopic study on the copper(II) binding mode of prion octapeptide and its pH dependence. Biochemistry. 35: 11560-11569.(1999)

135. Miura, T., A. Hori-i, and H. Takeuchi, Metal-dependent alpha-helix formation promoted by the glycine-rich octapeptide region of prion protein. FEBS Lett. 2-3: 248-252.(1996)

136. Moore, R.C., I.Y. Lee, G.L. Silverman, P.M. Harrison, R. Strome, C. Heinrich, A. Karunaratne, S.H. Pasternak, M.A. Chishti, Y. Liang, P. Mastrangelo, K. Wang, A.F. Smit, S. Katamine, G.A. Carlson, F.E. Cohen, S.B. Prusiner, D.W. Melton, P. Tremblay, L.E. Hood, and D. Westaway, Ataxia in prion protein (PrP)-deficient mice is associated with upregulation of the novel PrP-like protein doppel. J Mol Biol. 4: 797-817.(1999)

137. Morley, J.F. and R.I. Morimoto, Regulation of longevity in Caenorhabditis elegans by heat shock factor and molecular chaperones. Mol Biol Cell. 2: 657-664.(2004)

138. Moya, K.L., R. Hassig, C. Creminon, I. Laffont, and L. Di Giamberardino, Enhanced detection and retrograde axonal transport of PrPc in peripheral nerve. J Neurochem. 1: 155-160.(2004)

139. Mushegian, A.R., J.R. Garey, J. Martin, and L.X. Liu, Large-scale taxonomic profiling of eukaryotic model organisms: a comparison of orthologous proteins encoded by the human, fly, nematode, and yeast genomes. Genome Res. 6: 590-598.(1998)

140. Nishida, N., P. Tremblay, T. Sugimoto, K. Shigematsu, S. Shirabe, C. Petromilli, S.P. Erpel, R. Nakaoke, R. Atarashi, T. Houtani, M. Torchia, S. Sakaguchi, S.J. DeArmond, S.B. Prusiner, and S. Katamine, A mouse prion protein transgene rescues mice deficient for the prion protein gene from purkinje cell degeneration and demyelination. Lab Invest. 6: 689-697.(1999)

141. Oeda, T., S. Shimohama, N. Kitagawa, R. Kohno, T. Imura, H. Shibasaki, and N. Ishii, Oxidative stress causes abnormal accumulation of familial amyotrophic lateral sclerosis-related mutant SOD1 in transgenic Caenorhabditis elegans. Hum Mol Genet. 19: 2013-2023.(2001)

142. Oesch, B., D. Westaway, M. Walchli, M.P. McKinley, S.B. Kent, R. Aebersold, R.A. Barry, P. Tempst, D.B. Teplow, L.E. Hood, and et al., A cellular gene encodes scrapie PrP 27-30 protein. Cell. 4: 735-746.(1985)

143. Oh, S.W., A. Mukhopadhyay, N. Svrzikapa, F. Jiang, R.J. Davis, and H.A. Tissenbaum, JNK regulates lifespan in Caenorhabditis elegans by modulating nuclear translocation of forkhead transcription factor/DAF-16. Proc Natl Acad Sci U S A. 12: 4494-4499.(2005)

144. Pan, K.M., M. Baldwin, J. Nguyen, M. Gasset, A. Serban, D. Groth, I. Mehlhorn, Z. Huang, R.J. Fletterick, F.E. Cohen, and et al., Conversion of alpha-helices into beta-sheets features in the formation of the scrapie prion proteins. Proc Natl Acad Sci U S A. 23: 10962-10966.(1993)

145. Park, K.W. and L. Li, Cytoplasmic expression of mouse prion protein causes severe toxicity in Caenorhabditis elegans. Biochem Biophys Res Commun. 4: 697-702.(2008)

146. Pauly, P.C. and D.A. Harris, Copper stimulates endocytosis of the prion protein. J Biol Chem. 50: 33107-33110.(1998)

147. Perera, W.S. and N.M. Hooper, Ablation of the metal ion-induced endocytosis of the prion protein by disease-associated mutation of the octarepeat region. Curr Biol. 7: 519-523.(2001)

148. Pietri, M., A. Caprini, S. Mouillet-Richard, E. Pradines, M. Ermonval, J. Grassi, O. Kellermann, and B. Schneider, Overstimulation of PrPC signaling pathways by prion peptide 106-126 causes oxidative injury of bioaminergic neuronal cells. J Biol Chem. 38: 28470-28479.(2006)

149. Pirkkala, L., P. Nykanen, and L. Sistonen, Roles of the heat shock transcription factors in regulation of the heat shock response and beyond. Faseb J. 7: 1118-1131.(2001)

150. Prusiner, S.B., Novel proteinaceous infectious particles cause scrapie. Science. 4542: 136-144.(1982)

151. Prusiner, S.B., Molecular biology of prion diseases. Science. 5012: 1515-1522.(1991)

152. Prusiner, S.B., Prions. Proc Natl Acad Sci U S A. 23: 13363-13383.(1998)

153. Prusiner, S.B., D.C. Bolton, D.F. Groth, K.A. Bowman, S.P. Cochran, and M.P. McKinley, Further purification and characterization of scrapie prions. Biochemistry. 26: 6942-6950.(1982)

154. Prusiner, S.B., S.P. Cochran, D.F. Groth, D.E. Downey, K.A. Bowman, and H.M. Martinez, Measurement of the scrapie agent using an incubation time interval assay. Ann Neurol. 4: 353-358.(1982)
155. Prusiner, S.B., D.F. Groth, D.C. Bolton, S.B. Kent, and L.E. Hood, Purification and structural studies of a major scrapie prion protein. Cell. 1: 127-134.(1984)
156. Przybysz, A.J., K.P. Choe, L.J. Roberts, and K. Strange, Increased age reduces DAF-16 and SKN-1 signaling and the hormetic response of Caenorhabditis elegans to the xenobiotic juglone. Mech Ageing Dev. 6: 357-369.(2009)
157. Qin, K., D.S. Yang, Y. Yang, M.A. Chishti, L.J. Meng, H.A. Kretzschmar, C.M. Yip, P.E. Fraser, and D. Westaway, Copper(II)-induced conformational changes and protease resistance in recombinant and cellular PrP. Effect of protein age and deamidation. J Biol Chem. 25: 19121-19131.(2000)
158. Qin, K., L. Zhao, Y. Tang, S. Bhatta, J.M. Simard, and R.Y. Zhao, Doppel-induced apoptosis and counteraction by cellular prion protein in neuroblastoma and astrocytes. Neuroscience. 3: 1375-1388.(2006)
159. Quaglio, E., R. Chiesa, and D.A. Harris, Copper converts the cellular prion protein into a protease-resistant species that is distinct from the scrapie isoform. J Biol Chem. 14: 11432-11438.(2001)
160. Race, R., A. Raines, G.J. Raymond, B. Caughey, and B. Chesebro, Long-term subclinical carrier state precedes scrapie replication and adaptation in a resistant species: analogies to bovine spongiform encephalopathy and variant Creutzfeldt-Jakob disease in humans. J Virol. 21: 10106-10112.(2001)
161. Rachidi, W., A. Mange, A. Senator, P. Guiraud, J. Riondel, M. Benboubetra, A. Favier, and S. Lehmann, Prion infection impairs copper binding of cultured cells. J Biol Chem. 17: 14595-14598.(2003)
162. Rachidi, W., D. Vilette, P. Guiraud, M. Arlotto, J. Riondel, H. Laude, S. Lehmann, and A. Favier, Expression of prion protein increases cellular copper binding and antioxidant enzyme activities but not copper delivery. J Biol Chem. 11: 9064-9072.(2003)
163. Rae, T.D., P.J. Schmidt, R.A. Pufahl, V.C. Culotta, and T.V. O'Halloran, Undetectable intracellular free copper: the requirement of a copper chaperone for superoxide dismutase. Science. 5415: 805-808.(1999)
164. Rogers, M., A. Taraboulos, M. Scott, D. Groth, and S.B. Prusiner, Intracellular accumulation of the cellular prion protein after mutagenesis of its Asn-linked glycosylation sites. Glycobiology. 1: 101-109.(1990)

165. Roucou, X., P.N. Giannopoulos, Y. Zhang, J. Jodoin, C.G. Goodyer, and A. LeBlanc, Cellular prion protein inhibits proapoptotic Bax conformational change in human neurons and in breast carcinoma MCF-7 cells. Cell Death Differ. 7: 783-795.(2005)

166. Roucou, X., Q. Guo, Y. Zhang, C.G. Goodyer, and A.C. LeBlanc, Cytosolic prion protein is not toxic and protects against Bax-mediated cell death in human primary neurons. J Biol Chem. 42: 40877-40881.(2003)

167. Russell, S.J. and C.R. Kahn, Endocrine regulation of ageing. Nat Rev Mol Cell Biol. 9: 681-691.(2007)

168. Ryou, C., Prions and prion diseases: fundamentals and mechanistic details. J Microbiol Biotechnol. 7: 1059-1070.(2007)

169. Sakaguchi, S., S. Katamine, N. Nishida, R. Moriuchi, K. Shigematsu, T. Sugimoto, A. Nakatani, Y. Kataoka, T. Houtani, S. Shirabe, H. Okada, S. Hasegawa, T. Miyamoto, and T. Noda, Loss of cerebellar Purkinje cells in aged mice homozygous for a disrupted PrP gene. Nature. 6574: 528-531.(1996)

170. Sakudo, A., D.C. Lee, S. Li, T. Nakamura, Y. Matsumoto, K. Saeki, S. Itohara, K. Ikuta, and T. Onodera, PrP cooperates with STI1 to regulate SOD activity in PrP-deficient neuronal cell line. Biochem Biophys Res Commun. 1: 14-19.(2005)

171. Sakudo, A., I. Nakamura, S. Tsuji, and K. Ikuta, GPI-anchorless human prion protein is secreted and glycosylated but lacks superoxide dismutase activity. Int J Mol Med. 2: 217-222.(2008)

172. Sakurai-Yamashita, Y., S. Sakaguchi, D. Yoshikawa, N. Okimura, Y. Masuda, S. Katamine, and M. Niwa, Female-specific neuroprotection against transient brain ischemia observed in mice devoid of prion protein is abolished by ectopic expression of prion protein-like protein. Neuroscience. 1: 281-287.(2005)

173. Sampayo, J.N., M.S. Gill, and G.J. Lithgow, Oxidative stress and aging--the use of superoxide dismutase/catalase mimetics to extend lifespan. Biochem Soc Trans. Pt 6: 1305-1307.(2003)

174. Sampayo, J.N., A. Olsen, and G.J. Lithgow, Oxidative stress in Caenorhabditis elegans: protective effects of superoxide dismutase/catalase mimetics. Aging Cell. 6: 319-326.(2003)

175. Santuccione, A., V. Sytnyk, I. Leshchyns'ka, and M. Schachner, Prion protein recruits its neuronal receptor NCAM to lipid rafts to activate p59fyn and to enhance neurite outgrowth. J Cell Biol. 2: 341-354.(2005)

176. Schnabel, H. and R. Schnabel, An Organ-Specific Differentiation Gene, pha-1, from Caenorhabditis elegans. Science. 4981: 686-688.(1990)

177. Schneider, B., V. Mutel, M. Pietri, M. Ermonval, S. Mouillet-Richard, and O. Kellermann, NADPH oxidase and extracellular regulated kinases 1/2 are targets of prion protein signaling in neuronal and nonneuronal cells. Proc Natl Acad Sci U S A. 23: 13326-13331.(2003)

178. Shmerling, D., I. Hegyi, M. Fischer, T. Blattler, S. Brandner, J. Gotz, T. Rulicke, E. Flechsig, A. Cozzio, C. von Mering, C. Hangartner, A. Aguzzi, and C. Weissmann, Expression of amino-terminally truncated PrP in the mouse leading to ataxia and specific cerebellar lesions. Cell. 2: 203-214.(1998)

179. Sigurdsson, B., British Veterinary Journal: 341-354.(1954)

180. Silhavy, T.J. and J.R. Beckwith, Uses of lac fusions for the study of biological problems. Microbiol Rev. 4: 398-418.(1985)

181. Singh, V. and A. Aballay, Heat-shock transcription factor (HSF)-1 pathway required for Caenorhabditis elegans immunity. Proc Natl Acad Sci U S A. 35: 13092-13097.(2006)

182. Singh, V. and A. Aballay, Heat shock and genetic activation of HSF-1 enhance immunity to bacteria. Cell Cycle. 21: 2443-2446.(2006)

183. Smith, P.K., R.I. Krohn, G.T. Hermanson, A.K. Mallia, F.H. Gartner, M.D. Provenzano, E.K. Fujimoto, N.M. Goeke, B.J. Olson, and D.C. Klenk, Measurement of protein using bicinchoninic acid. Anal Biochem. 1: 76-85.(1985)

184. Spector, D. and R. Goldman, Constructing and Expressing GFP Fusion Proteins. Living Cell Imaging. New York: Cold Spring Harbor Laboratory Press.(2005)

185. Spraker, T.R., M.W. Miller, E.S. Williams, D.M. Getzy, W.J. Adrian, G.G. Schoonveld, R.A. Spowart, K.I. O'Rourke, J.M. Miller, and P.A. Merz, Spongiform encephalopathy in free-ranging mule deer (Odocoileus hemionus), white-tailed deer (Odocoileus virginianus) and Rocky Mountain elk (Cervus elaphus nelsoni) in northcentral Colorado. J Wildl Dis. 1: 1-6.(1997)

186. Spudich, A., R. Frigg, E. Kilic, U. Kilic, B. Oesch, A. Raeber, C.L. Bassetti, and D.M. Hermann, Aggravation of ischemic brain injury by prion protein deficiency: role of ERK-1/-2 and STAT-1. Neurobiol Dis. 2: 442-449.(2005)

187. Stahl, N., D.R. Borchelt, K. Hsiao, and S.B. Prusiner, Scrapie prion protein contains a phosphatidylinositol glycolipid. Cell. 2: 229-240.(1987)

188. Steele, A.D., J.G. Emsley, P.H. Ozdinler, S. Lindquist, and J.D. Macklis, Prion protein (PrPc) positively regulates neural precursor proliferation during developmental and adult mammalian neurogenesis. Proc Natl Acad Sci U S A. 9: 3416-3421.(2006)

189. Steinacker, P., P. Schwarz, K. Reim, P. Brechlin, O. Jahn, H. Kratzin, A. Aitken, J. Wiltfang, A. Aguzzi, E. Bahn, H.C. Baxter, N. Brose, and M. Otto, Unchanged survival

rates of 14-3-3gamma knockout mice after inoculation with pathological prion protein. Mol Cell Biol. 4: 1339-1346.(2005)
190. Stender, A., Spastische Pseudosklerose Jakobs. ZEITSCHRIFT FUR DIE GESAMTE NEUROLOGIE UND PSYCHIATRIE: 528-543.(1930)
191. Stiernagle, T., Maintenance of C. elegans. C. elegans - A Practical Approach, ed. I.A. Hope. Oxford: Oxford University Press. p. 57-67.(2005)
192. Stockel, J., J. Safar, A.C. Wallace, F.E. Cohen, and S.B. Prusiner, Prion protein selectively binds copper(II) ions. Biochemistry. 20: 7185-7193.(1998)
193. Sulston, J. and J. Hodgkin, The Nematode Caenorhabditis elegans, ed. W.B. Wood. New York: Cold Spring Harbor Laboratory Press. p. 586-588.(1988)
194. Sulston, J.E., D.G. Albertson, and J.N. Thomson, The Caenorhabditis elegans male: postembryonic development of nongonadal structures. Dev Biol. 2: 542-576.(1980)
195. Sulston, J.E., E. Schierenberg, J.G. White, and J.N. Thomson, The embryonic cell lineage of the nematode Caenorhabditis elegans. Dev Biol. 1: 64-119.(1983)
196. Sunyach, C., M.A. Cisse, C.A. da Costa, B. Vincent, and F. Checler, The C-terminal products of cellular prion protein processing, C1 and C2, exert distinct influence on p53-dependent staurosporine-induced caspase-3 activation. J Biol Chem. 3: 1956-1963.(2007)
197. Sunyach, C., A. Jen, J. Deng, K.T. Fitzgerald, Y. Frobert, J. Grassi, M.W. McCaffrey, and R. Morris, The mechanism of internalization of glycosylphosphatidylinositol-anchored prion protein. Embo J. 14: 3591-3601.(2003)
198. Swain, S.C., K. Keusekotten, R. Baumeister, and S.R. Sturzenbaum, C. elegans metallothioneins: new insights into the phenotypic effects of cadmium toxicosis. J Mol Biol. 4: 951-959.(2004)
199. Tawe, W.N., M.L. Eschbach, R.D. Walter, and K. Henkle-Duhrsen, Identification of stress-responsive genes in Caenorhabditis elegans using RT-PCR differential display. Nucleic Acids Res. 7: 1621-1627.(1998)
200. Taylor, D.R. and N.M. Hooper, The prion protein and lipid rafts. Mol Membr Biol. 1: 89-99.(2006)
201. Taylor, D.R., N.T. Watt, W.S. Perera, and N.M. Hooper, Assigning functions to distinct regions of the N-terminus of the prion protein that are involved in its copper-stimulated, clathrin-dependent endocytosis. J Cell Sci. Pt 21: 5141-5153.(2005)
202. Tobler, I., T. Deboer, and M. Fischer, Sleep and sleep regulation in normal and prion protein-deficient mice. J Neurosci. 5: 1869-1879.(1997)

203. Tobler, I., S.E. Gaus, T. Deboer, P. Achermann, M. Fischer, T. Rulicke, M. Moser, B. Oesch, P.A. McBride, and J.C. Manson, Altered circadian activity rhythms and sleep in mice devoid of prion protein. Nature. 6575: 639-642.(1996)
204. Triarhou, L.C., Josef Gerstmann (1887-1969). J Neurol. 4: 614-615.(2008)
205. Tullet, J.M., M. Hertweck, J.H. An, J. Baker, J.Y. Hwang, S. Liu, R.P. Oliveira, R. Baumeister, and T.K. Blackwell, Direct inhibition of the longevity-promoting factor SKN-1 by insulin-like signaling in C. elegans. Cell. 6: 1025-1038.(2008)
206. van Delft, M.F. and D.C. Huang, How the Bcl-2 family of proteins interact to regulate apoptosis. Cell Res. 2: 203-213.(2006)
207. Van Remmen, H., Y. Ikeno, M. Hamilton, M. Pahlavani, N. Wolf, S.R. Thorpe, N.L. Alderson, J.W. Baynes, C.J. Epstein, T.T. Huang, J. Nelson, R. Strong, and A. Richardson, Life-long reduction in MnSOD activity results in increased DNA damage and higher incidence of cancer but does not accelerate aging. Physiol Genomics. 1: 29-37.(2003)
208. Vanfleteren, J.R., In Nematodes as Biological Models, ed. B.M. Zuckermann. Vol. 2 New York: Academic Press. p. 47-49.(1980)
209. Varela-Nallar, L., E.M. Toledo, M.A. Chacon, and N.C. Inestrosa, The functional links between prion protein and copper. Biol Res. 1: 39-44.(2006)
210. Varela-Nallar, L., E.M. Toledo, L.F. Larrondo, A.L. Cabral, V.R. Martins, and N.C. Inestrosa, Induction of cellular prion protein gene expression by copper in neurons. Am J Physiol Cell Physiol. 1: C271-281.(2006)
211. Vassallo, N. and J. Herms, Cellular prion protein function in copper homeostasis and redox signalling at the synapse. J Neurochem. 3: 538-544.(2003)
212. Viles, J.H., F.E. Cohen, S.B. Prusiner, D.B. Goodin, P.E. Wright, and H.J. Dyson, Copper binding to the prion protein: structural implications of four identical cooperative binding sites. Proc Natl Acad Sci U S A. 5: 2042-2047.(1999)
213. Viles, J.H., M. Klewpatinond, and R.C. Nadal, Copper and the structural biology of the prion protein. Biochem Soc Trans. Pt 6: 1288-1292.(2008)
214. Villanueva, A., J. Lozano, A. Morales, X. Lin, X. Deng, M.O. Hengartner, and R.N. Kolesnick, jkk-1 and mek-1 regulate body movement coordination and response to heavy metals through jnk-1 in Caenorhabditis elegans. Embo J. 18: 5114-5128.(2001)
215. Viswanathan, M., S.K. Kim, A. Berdichevsky, and L. Guarente, A role for SIR-2.1 regulation of ER stress response genes in determining C. elegans life span. Dev Cell. 5: 605-615.(2005)

216. Waggoner, D.J., B. Drisaldi, T.B. Bartnikas, R.L. Casareno, J.R. Prohaska, J.D. Gitlin, and D.A. Harris, Brain copper content and cuproenzyme activity do not vary with prion protein expression level. J Biol Chem. 11: 7455-7458.(2000)

217. Walter, E.D., M. Chattopadhyay, and G.L. Millhauser, The affinity of copper binding to the prion protein octarepeat domain: evidence for negative cooperativity. Biochemistry. 43: 13083-13092.(2006)

218. Weinkove, D., J.R. Halstead, D. Gems, and N. Divecha, Long-term starvation and ageing induce AGE-1/PI 3-kinase-dependent translocation of DAF-16/FOXO to the cytoplasm. BMC Biol: 1.(2006)

219. Weise, J., R. Sandau, S. Schwarting, O. Crome, A. Wrede, W. Schulz-Schaeffer, I. Zerr, and M. Bahr, Deletion of cellular prion protein results in reduced Akt activation, enhanced postischemic caspase-3 activation, and exacerbation of ischemic brain injury. Stroke. 5: 1296-1300.(2006)

220. Wells, M.A., G.S. Jackson, S. Jones, L.L. Hosszu, C.J. Craven, A.R. Clarke, J. Collinge, and J.P. Waltho, A reassessment of copper(II) binding in the full-length prion protein. Biochem J. 3: 435-444.(2006)

221. Wells, M.A., C. Jelinska, L.L. Hosszu, C.J. Craven, A.R. Clarke, J. Collinge, J.P. Waltho, and G.S. Jackson, Multiple forms of copper (II) co-ordination occur throughout the disordered N-terminal region of the prion protein at pH 7.4. Biochem J. 3: 501-510.(2006)

222. Westergard, L., H.M. Christensen, and D.A. Harris, The cellular prion protein (PrP(C)): its physiological function and role in disease. Biochim Biophys Acta. 6: 629-644.(2007)

223. White, A.R., S.J. Collins, F. Maher, M.F. Jobling, L.R. Stewart, J.M. Thyer, K. Beyreuther, C.L. Masters, and R. Cappai, Prion protein-deficient neurons reveal lower glutathione reductase activity and increased susceptibility to hydrogen peroxide toxicity. Am J Pathol. 5: 1723-1730.(1999)

224. White, A.R., G. Multhaup, D. Galatis, W.J. McKinstry, M.W. Parker, R. Pipkorn, K. Beyreuther, C.L. Masters, and R. Cappai, Contrasting, species-dependent modulation of copper-mediated neurotoxicity by the Alzheimer's disease amyloid precursor protein. J Neurosci. 2: 365-376.(2002)

225. White, J.G., E. Southgate, J.N. Thomson, and S. Brenner, The structure of the nervous system of the nematode Caenorhabditis elegans. Phil. Trans. Royal Soc. London. Series B, Biol Scien. 1165 (Nov. 12, 1986): 1-340.(1986)

226. Whittal, R.M., H.L. Ball, F.E. Cohen, A.L. Burlingame, S.B. Prusiner, and M.A. Baldwin, Copper binding to octarepeat peptides of the prion protein monitored by mass spectrometry. Protein Sci. 2: 332-343.(2000)

227. Wiggins, R.C., Prion stability and infectivity in the environment. Neurochem Res. 1: 158-168.(2009)
228. Wong, B.S., T. Liu, R. Li, T. Pan, R.B. Petersen, M.A. Smith, P. Gambetti, G. Perry, J.C. Manson, D.R. Brown, and M.S. Sy, Increased levels of oxidative stress markers detected in the brains of mice devoid of prion protein. J Neurochem. 2: 565-572.(2001)
229. Wong, B.S., C. Venien-Bryan, R.A. Williamson, D.R. Burton, P. Gambetti, M.S. Sy, D.R. Brown, and I.M. Jones, Copper refolding of prion protein. Biochem Biophys Res Commun. 3: 1217-1224.(2000)
230. Yanase, S., A. Onodera, P. Tedesco, T.E. Johnson, and N. Ishii, SOD-1 deletions in Caenorhabditis elegans alter the localization of intracellular reactive oxygen species and show molecular compensation. J Gerontol A Biol Sci Med Sci. 5: 530-539.(2009)
231. Yanase, S., K. Yasuda, and N. Ishii, Adaptive responses to oxidative damage in three mutants of Caenorhabditis elegans (age-1, mev-1 and daf-16) that affect life span. Mech Ageing Dev. 12: 1579-1587.(2002)
232. Yang, W., J. Li, and S. Hekimi, A Measurable increase in oxidative damage due to reduction in superoxide detoxification fails to shorten the life span of long-lived mitochondrial mutants of Caenorhabditis elegans. Genetics. 4: 2063-2074.(2007)
233. Zanata, S.M., M.H. Lopes, A.F. Mercadante, G.N. Hajj, L.B. Chiarini, R. Nomizo, A.R. Freitas, A.L. Cabral, K.S. Lee, M.A. Juliano, E. de Oliveira, S.G. Jachieri, A. Burlingame, L. Huang, R. Linden, R.R. Brentani, and V.R. Martins, Stress-inducible protein 1 is a cell surface ligand for cellular prion that triggers neuroprotection. Embo J. 13: 3307-3316.(2002)
234. Zanusso, G., G. Vattemi, S. Ferrari, M. Tabaton, E. Pecini, T. Cavallaro, G. Tomelleri, M. Filosto, P. Tonin, E. Nardelli, N. Rizzuto, and S. Monaco, Increased expression of the normal cellular isoform of prion protein in inclusion-body myositis, inflammatory myopathies and denervation atrophy. Brain Pathol. 2: 182-189.(2001)
235. Zeng, F., N.T. Watt, A.R. Walmsley, and N.M. Hooper, Tethering the N-terminus of the prion protein compromises the cellular response to oxidative stress. J Neurochem. 3: 480-490.(2003)
236. Zhang, Y., X. Zhao, and P.Y. Wang, Molecular dynamics study of the fibril elongation of the prion protein fragment PrP106-126. J Theor Biol. 2: 238-242.(2007)
237. Zomosa-Signoret, V., J.D. Arnaud, P. Fontes, M.T. Alvarez-Martinez, and J.P. Liautard, Physiological role of the cellular prion protein. Vet Res. 4: 9.(2008)

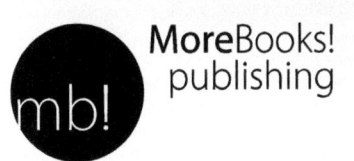

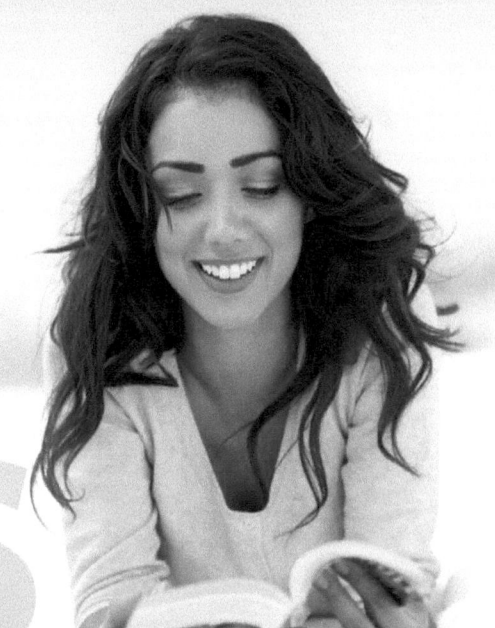

i want morebooks!

Buy your books fast and straightforward online - at one of world's fastest growing online book stores! Environmentally sound due to Print-on-Demand technologies.

Buy your books online at

www.get-morebooks.com

Kaufen Sie Ihre Bücher schnell und unkompliziert online – auf einer der am schnellsten wachsenden Buchhandelsplattformen weltweit! Dank Print-On-Demand umwelt- und ressourcenschonend produziert.

Bücher schneller online kaufen

www.morebooks.de

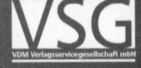

VDM Verlagsservicegesellschaft mbH
Heinrich-Böcking-Str. 6-8　　Telefon: +49 681 3720 174　　info@vdm-vsg.de
D - 66121 Saarbrücken　　Telefax: +49 681 3720 1749　　www.vdm-vsg.de

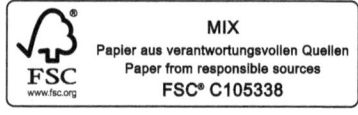

Printed by Books on Demand GmbH, Norderstedt / Germany